# Speech and Language
# Clinical Process and Practice

# Speech and Language Clinical Process and Practice

MONICA BRAY, ALISON ROSS
*Speech and Language Sciences Group,*
*Leeds Metropolitan University*

CELIA TODD
*Speech and Language Therapist, Trecare NHS Trust,*
*formerly of Leeds Metropolitan University*

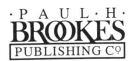

·P A U L·H·
BROOKES
PUBLISHING CO

Baltimore • Toronto

© 1999 Whurr Publishers Ltd
First published 1999 by
Whurr Publishers Ltd
19b Compton Terrace, London N1 2UN, England

Reprinted 1999, 2000, 2002 and 2003

**British Library Cataloguing in Publication Data**
A catalogue record for this book is available from the British
Library.

ISBN 186156 094 X

Printed and bound in the UK by Athenæum Press Ltd,
Gateshead, Tyne & Wear

# Contents

# Preface

This book grew out of our own professional development as speech and language clinicians and our work with speech and language therapy students. Our experiences with students in clinical settings, workshops, seminars, tutorials and lectures have led us to an understanding of the struggles encountered and the questions asked by individuals who are in the transitional state from student to qualified clinician. The only way to be ready to face the demands of professional practice and life-long learning is thoroughly to understand the process and practice of clinical work.

The book is primarily for students, whom we have addressed throughout the text and considered when attempting to highlight the experiences and feelings they may encounter. But we also hope that it will be of value to others who work with students, and that some aspects of the book may be appreciated by experienced clinicians as an opportunity to revisit what is involved in therapy and professional practice. From feedback received when we have discussed the book with others, we suggest that it may provide in particular a source of information for those just starting in the profession or returning to it after a time away. It is not intended to teach clinical skills or core knowledge, but to provide a combination of information, ideas, case illustrations and concepts that we hope will guide students' professional practice. The ideas presented draw on the authors' range of reading, experience and thinking over many years, and represent our approaches and beliefs. It would be surprising if all clinicians agreed with everything we say, and where disagreement arises, this should provide the focus for healthy debate.

As the text does not attempt to provide a background of knowledge about speech pathology and therapy, linguistics, medical sciences, audiology, education, psychology or any of the many fields of theory that are important to the speech and language clinician, students are advised to use this book in tandem with their other learning experiences. We have concentrated on the areas that apply all of this learning and help to link theory and therapy to the clinical process and professional practice.

Clinical process is about the methods and actions used to effect positive change in people's communication functioning. Students commonly yearn to be told what to do when faced with a clinical problem. While demonstrating and explaining techniques such as ways of administering assessments, ways of interacting, and ways of shaping and reinforcing behaviours is essential, the appropriate and successful use of such methods must depend on a wealth of awareness, knowledge, attitudes and behaviours. It is these that we have tried to capture in this book.

Professional practice is about the context of our work, the people with whom we work, and the standards, attitudes and behaviours we adopt as clinicians in order to provide a high quality of care for people with communication disorders. This book endeavours to review the scope of speech and language practice.

The first two chapters set the scene by discussing the speech and language clinician and the nature of intervention in general. Chapters 3 and 4 give the reader a chance to consider in depth the actual processes and practices that take place when clinician and client come together. Chapters 5 and 6 take a broader perspective, encouraging reflection on the role of the speech and language clinician in more detail. The place of and need for paperwork to support clinical practice is discussed in Chapter 7, and finally, in Chapter 8, we look at the transition from student to qualified clinician and the nature of continuing professional development. We would encourage students to read the book from cover to cover, but each chapter also stands alone, allowing readers to make choices about where they wish to focus. The many case discussions found through the book are based not on actual individuals but on an amalgamation of clients we have known through our many years of clinical practice.

While we acknowledge that speech and language clinicians may be male or female, we found that our initial attempts to signal this by he/she, his/her inhibited the flow for the reader, and therefore where gender has to be indicated, the female form has been chosen.

In learning we move from stage to stage, building on what we know, and moving from vague and uncertain formulations to clearer and more precise awareness. Readers will come to this book from different starting points, bringing with them their own personal knowledge and experience. We hope it will enable them to move forward to a greater understanding of what goes on in clinical work.

Teaching and learning are two sides of the same coin. As we teach students, so we learn from them, thus expanding and increasing our own knowledge, skills and attitudes. This book is therefore dedicated to all our students past, present and future from whom we have learned so much and through whom we hope to continue to develop.

*Monica Bray*
*Alison Ross*
*Celia Todd*
July 1998

# Chapter 1
# The Speech and Language Clinician

Prior to unravelling the mysteries of the processes, procedures, relationships and activities involved in managing communication disorders, it is helpful to take some time to consider the characteristics and roles of the professionals who are central to this field. These are the people who, in this book, we have chosen to call speech and language clinicians. To build up a picture of these people we will try to answer a few questions about their work:

- What is the focus and range of their work?
- Where do they work?
- Who do they help?
- What approaches are applied in their work?
- What knowledge, skills and attitudes are special to their work?

The following is only intended as an introduction to the more comprehensive discussion that follows later in the book.

## Focus and range of the work of the speech and language clinician

'Logopedist', 'speech-language pathologist', 'speech pathologist', 'speech-language pathologist and audiologist', 'speech and language therapist', 'orthophonist', 'phonoaudiologist', 'speech therapist', 'speech clinician' and 'communication clinician' are some of the titles, or the English translations of titles, that are used by various nations (ASHA and IALP, 1994) to denote a professional who is specifically qualified to work with individuals or groups of people who have speech and language disorders. In reality, the work will not be restricted to a narrow focus on speech and language, but will encompass wider aspects of human communication as well as the functions and processes that are related to speech and language, such as swallowing and hearing.

1

Cultural, political, financial, education and training, employment and other national differences mean the emphasis of the work practice of speech and language clinicians varies from country to country. In some countries, speech and language clinicians concentrate on children with speech and language disorders, including those disorders that are secondary to deafness and special education; in others the work is hospital-based and concerns disorders associated with medical conditions. In some countries the work involves both child and adult disorders in schools, hospitals and other settings. Sometimes the speech and language clinician will be qualified in another field as well, such as audiology and hearing therapy, special education, or another rehabilitation specialism, such as physiotherapy, occupational therapy or ophthalmology (Lesser, 1992). The methods that speech and language clinicians use, including the degree of formality in their methods, will also differ. There is, however, a great deal of common ground between speech and language clinicians in their commitment to the prevention, assessment, intervention, management and scientific study of communication and associated disorders. Although this book is likely to have a British bias, we will endeavour to refer to a range of practices that will be familiar to, or can be readily applied in, other nations.

## Speech and language clinical contexts

*Clinician* is the most universally appropriate term to describe the manner of work of the specialist who provides care for people with speech and language and related problems. It is selected in preference to 'pathologist', which implies a study of disorder or disease without intervention, or 'therapist', which suggests a concentration on treatment. The term clinician may conjure up images of work in medical settings, either at the hospital bedside or in health clinics, and a primary concern for presenting conditions and disorders. However, most importantly, it conveys the message that the specialist concerned is objective and applies a scientific, problem-solving approach to the observation, evaluation and management of people – the *clients*.

As a speech and language clinician you may work in hospital wards and hospital or health centre clinics, but there are other places where you can contact clients. You might make contact at their place of residence, perhaps the family home or a care home, or in the place they go to in the daytime, such as a day centre or school. You may also work in other settings, including resource centres that provide a service for augmentative communication system users. To help answer the question 'Where do they work?', the Royal College of Speech and Language Therapists has compiled a list of settings or service locations (RCSLT, 1996), which is presented below. From this you should gain a sense of the breadth of the possible contexts of client-related work:

- acute
- long-stay hospitals
- rehabilitation centres
- community clinics
- specialist outpatient centres
- day centres – including adult training centres, social education centres and resource centres
- supported living or group homes
- domiciliary (i.e. visits to the home of the client)
- day nurseries
- child development centres
- mainstream schools
- special schools – including classes and units
- language units – including schools and classes
- nursery schools.

There is a range of types of organization in which speech and language clinicians are employed, in both this and other countries. Among the many possible employment settings for speech and language clinicians are:

- public sector organizations, such as a national health service or a social or welfare service
- individual or group private practice
- voluntary sector organizations funded by grants and charities, for example for the visually or hearing impaired, the brain injured, or specifically for people with communication disorders.

Although working practices may vary according to the requirements of the employing organization, you will find that the values shared and practised by speech and language clinicians are fundamentally the same.

## The speech and language client

Speech and language clinicians are concerned with *individuals* and groups of individuals, and their abilities in communication and related areas such as swallowing and hearing. The use of the term 'client' rather than 'patient' is chosen to avoid any implication that the person concerned is ill or has a medical condition, or that the treatment given should be merely symptom-related. This means that there is an acknowledgement that problems such as the strained voice of a teacher or the delayed language development of a child may have little or no association with a medical condition. Further, that each of these cases may require intervention that goes beyond instruction related to the observed impairment, i.e. in vocal exercises for the teacher or in language production tasks for the child. The intervention is likely instead to be based on changing underlying influences such as environment, listening skills or attitudes.

There is no intention to ignore the fact that many speech and language clients do have a communication problem resulting from a medical condition, such as Parkinson's disease, stroke, head injury, cerebral palsy, hearing loss, cleft palate or laryngectomy. These people will need the support of medical personnel. However, each of these people is far more than the outcome of a medical problem. They have different backgrounds, values and attitudes, experiences, physical characteristics and behaviours, and all these factors, as well as their medical condition, will contribute to the way in which the individual deals with his or her ability to communicate. This should be accounted for in the management decisions of medical and other personnel. The client should not be viewed merely as a part of a medical problem, and should not be treated just like the last person who presented with the same diagnosis.

The choice of the term client rather than patient also places the individual with the communication problem in an active rather than passive role in the relationship with the clinician and the speech and language service provided. In the world of business, 'client' is often used interchangeably with 'customer', 'consumer' and 'user' (Harrow and Shaw, 1992). Implicit in this group of words are concepts of financial exchange in return for a product or service, and of the rights and demands of the individual, and their freedom to go elsewhere. These concepts similarly underpin care provision, including speech and language services. Whether as a third party payer, through a national health or private insurance scheme, or as a more direct purchaser, the client pays and is therefore a customer as well as a user and consumer of the service. The client has choices to indicate his or her preferences and to take or leave the care that is offered (Kineen, 1994). It is this business-oriented perspective, as well as a personal and professional dimension of clinical relationships and intervention, that leads the clinician to establish mutually agreed contracts with her clients, in which all clients have equal rights to be provided with the best possible quality of care and to be involved in management decisions. This is considered further in the discussion of the client-centred approach, below.

## Speech and language disorder classification

While never losing sight of the individuality of each client, for convenience, speech and language clinicians tend to classify communication disorders according to the presenting problem. This involves broad categories, such as *developmental*, indicating that the problem has been present in some way since infancy, *acquired*, indicating that the onset of the problem was after infancy, or *progressive*, indicating a deterioration associated with either a developmental or an acquired condition. There have been several attempts to categorize the many and varied types of communication and related disorders that can occur. Two classification systems are given below.

*1. Classification of presenting disorders (Royal College of Speech and Language Therapists, 1996)*

- Acquired language disorder/adult aphasia
- Acquired childhood aphasia
- Developmental speech and language disorders
- Written language disorders
     (a) developmental
     (b) acquired
- Developmental dysarthria
- Acquired dysarthria
- Acquired phonetic disorders
- Dysphonia
- Dysfluency
- Dysphagia
- Eating and drinking difficulties in children

*2. Classification of linguistic pathologies (Crystal and Varley, 1993)*

- Cognitive disorders, e.g. thought disorders, autism and learning difficulties
- Language disorders, e.g. aphasia, and developmental language disorder
- Apraxia
- Dysarthria
- Disorders of voice, e.g. vocal abuse and laryngectomy
- Disorders of articulation, e.g. cleft palate and glossectomy
- Hearing impairment
- Agnosia

# Approaches applied in speech and language clinical practice

In the earlier discussion of the choice of use of the term client, it was noted that speech and language clinicians do not adopt a narrow symptom-based approach to practice. Instead it is agreed that a *holistic* approach is essential in the assessment and intervention of communication problems. Not only should the clinician endeavour to address any voice, fluency, speech and language, or swallowing problem that presents, but she must consider the wider effects and implications of the problem.

Communication and related disorders can lead to a loss of independence, a change in lifestyle, confusion, frustration, failure at school, adverse reactions from others and difficulty with relationships. As the disorder will normally be greater than the sum of the presenting features, the clinician needs to look at every contributing factor and determine the wide-ranging intervention that could help to alleviate the disorder. Management decisions should be based on a wealth of knowledge about the person, the problem complex, the communication experience and needs of the individual, and, not least, his or her wishes for change. The following examples illustrate how decision making is based on more than the overt features or the disorder classification:

1.  An adult with a decline in written language skills following stroke who had never previously achieved or needed high-level literacy skills would not be expected to contemplate more than the simplest reading and writing task.
2.  A person who stammers and is comfortable with his or her image of self and disfluent speech would not be a candidate for therapy.
3.  A child with a language delay who is teased at school or whose parents are overanxious and inappropriately correcting disordered speech attempts might be given higher priority than a child who does not have to cope with the added problems.

A client-centred, non-directive approach to therapy, first put forward by Rogers in the 1940s (Rogers, 1951), is advocated by most speech and language clinicians and will be promoted in this book. This does not mean that more directed approaches will not be considered. Unlike directive approaches, where the role of the clinician or therapist applies rather prescribed methods to achieve change, the client-centred approach emphasizes the role of the therapist as a *facilitator*. The therapist, in this case the speech and language clinician, encourages clients to:

*   explore aspects of themselves and ways of relating to others
*   practise new behaviours
*   change their perceptions, attitudes and performance.

Throughout this process of development, reformulation and change, the speech and language clinician works in partnership with the client. As a speech and language clinician, you will draw on professional knowledge and skills to guide the collection of evidence, inform, clarify and provide the opportunity for the client to practise different behaviours. Additionally, you will offer a context of trust and empathy within which the client is *empowered*. This means that he or she adopts a sense of owner-ship of the therapy process and shares the responsibility for the outcomes. Thus we have an approach in which clinical decisions are a joint venture between the client and the clinician. The approach stresses the impor-tance of negotiation and choice, including choice about whether or not to receive treatment and choice about the direction of treatment.

Of particular importance in helping the client to effect change is the role of the clinician in listening, demystifying and clarifying. This involves attending to the person's view of him or herself, taking account of all the factors contributing to the disorder, and explaining and helping him or her to appreciate the nature of the problems, the alternative ways of addressing them and the prognosis or outcomes to expect from the choices made.

Implicit in this therapy approach, and a general underpinning principle of speech and language clinicians, is that the intended outcomes of therapy constitute positive change not 'cure'. As Finkelstein (1993) reminds us, the concept of cure is determined by standards and beliefs about what is normal. Speech and language clinicians do not seek to cure. They aim to offer optimal help in changing behaviours and attitudes within the boundaries appropriate for the individual, and to enable the client to attain the best quality of life he or she can within their own normality. This may be particularly difficult to come to terms with for some clients. A man who has an acquired disability, such as dysarthria following a head injury, may have a previous construct of self that he aspires to rebuild. A mother may expect her child who has learning difficulties to achieve the same level of language functioning as children of the same age who do not have learning difficulties. These situations will require a sensitive response and carefully managed support from the clinician.

It is not too difficult to appreciate how the client-centred approach works for adults who possess a reasonable level of cognitive skills and can comprehend and express ideas, consider alternatives, analyse and problem solve. But what happens in the case of a person who has severe linguistic impairment, learning difficulties or cognitive deficit, or who is an infant? In these cases a parent, relative, friend or, where none of these are available, a professional or other person, might be called upon to act as a proxy or advocate for the client. As Brechin and Swain (1988) explain, advocacy is based on the principle of creating opportunities for self-determination, that is, the power to make a decision for oneself. Within formal structures or informally, the advocate has responsibility for promoting decisions that will enable the client to have greater autonomy. Decisions should not be based on what might be easiest for, or preferred by, a carer, service or other agency. In this way, the advocate who contributes to speech and language management decisions should be the voice of the client.

### Professional judgement

In addition to the role of the client in determining the change that should be brought about, there are two other essential ingredients in the decision-making process that must be noted. These are the professional judgement of the speech and language clinician and the availability of provision and resources (Leahy, 1989).

*The professional judgement of the speech and language clinician*

While the preferences of the individual client have a high priority, decisions must be made in the light of what is realistic and possible in terms of theoretical and clinical knowledge. Speech and language theory and practice is an ever-growing body of understanding, supported by research and evidence of efficacy for particular intervention strategies. At the same time, the experience of each clinician will bring boundless evidence of practice that is appropriate and of value to clients.

*The availability of provision and resources*

Every service will have limits to its resources. This will affect how much time you can spend with clients, when you can spend the time and the type of intervention you can offer. You can only offer what is possible within the resources available and in your power to provide, but also, whatever you offer must be given in fairness to other service users. You cannot merely respond to demand and, while listening to and remaining in touch with the client, it is important not to overpromise (Kineen, 1994).

**Public promotion**

As Byers-Brown and Gilbert (1989) remind us, communication handicap is a product of the whole community, not only of the individual who has the disorder. A person with a communication problem is part of a social context within which both the individual and the community react and adapt in a variety of ways. To reduce the occurrence and effects of handicap, people who are likely to interact with individuals with potential and actual handicap need to be targeted. To this end another aspect of the work of speech and language clinicians is that of promoting public understanding of communication problems and people who have communication problems. In addition to responding to general opportunities to increase the knowledge and understanding of the population at large, clinicians might focus on selected groups who have contact with people with communication disorder. For example by:

- providing a series of talks and leading discussions with sets of children in their schools
- running workshops for staff of care homes for the elderly.

In these cases the client is not a specific person but a population group that is affected or at risk of being affected by communication disorder.

  The aim of the speech and language clinician is to provide 'the best possible care for those who suffer from communication handicap' (Byers-Brown and Gilbert, 1989). To achieve this diagnostic assessment, remedy, support, information and guidance have to be made available for the benefit of both those who 'suffer' and those who care for them. The key words explaining this management process are *assessment, treatment* and *advice or information*. These are not separate entities, as later chapters will explain, but interdependent aspects of the clinical process.

Constant *hypothesis testing*, that is, making and verifying tentative propositions, is central to the assessment, treatment, and advice and information-giving involved in clinical management. For example:

- You might observe that a child is uncommunicative in the clinic and so put forward a hypothesis that they are uncommunicative in other situations. You can then test this hypothesis by asking the mother or teacher about communication in the home and school, or by observing the child outside the clinic setting.
- You might form a hypothesis that a young child's language skills would improve if therapy concentrated on working with the mother. You can then introduce a programme involving the mother and later assess whether change has occurred.
- You might hypothesize that an adult's language deficit is exacerbated by a hearing loss. Following referral for audiometric assessment and subsequent fitting of a hearing aid you can monitor any improvement in language to test your hypothesis.

In this way, you explore the communication problem and the needs of the individual, you assess whether intervention is required and what intervention would be most appropriate, and then evaluate the degree to which the range of aspects of your intervention has achieved what you and the client intended.

## Knowledge, skills and attitudes of speech and language clinicians

What do these clinicians do that is special? You will not be the only professionals involved with people with disorders of communication. A schoolteacher helps children with reading, writing or spoken language problems. A teacher of the deaf helps children to compensate for their poor communication. A psychologist offers guidance to the parents of children with autism. A doctor advises people about their voice disorder. A nurse helps with the feeding problems arising from neurological disorder. A volunteer visitor offers a person who is language-impaired following a stroke support and practice in speech, comprehension, reading and writing. A care assistant encourages the communication skills of the elderly in a care home.

In spite of the contributions of others, it is only a speech and language clinician who is enabled through a range of learning and professional and practice development to bring together a particular set of knowledge, attitudes and skills that none of these people has, or indeed would need to or wish to acquire. At the same time, the speech and language clinician will be dependent on the different specialist sets of knowledge and skills of these experts. They will work together (see Chapter 5) to optimize the change in communication that we hope our clients will achieve.

There are four main disciplines at the core of our learning as speech and language clinicians – psychology, medical sciences, linguistics, and speech and language pathology. Additionally, you will draw on learning from many other fields, including education and sociology. The knowledge, skills and attitudes required by speech and language clinicians are accumulated through reading, listening and discussion, and through observation and practice. The learning of speech and language clinicians encompasses for example:

- human behaviour and how people perceive and learn
- language, language use and language development
- interpersonal skills, attitudes and reactions
- development from embryo to old age
- multicultural society and the policies that govern society
- anatomy and physiology, and medical conditions
- disorders of communication and their management.

The skills we need to acquire are equally far-ranging, e.g. planning, negotiating, assessment, explaining, observing, decision making, teaching, counselling and record keeping. The clinician also needs to develop and refine attitudes, including enthusiasm, adaptability, empathy, reliability and willingness to promote the needs of clients. This does not mean that other professionals and non-professionals do not apply some of the knowledge, skills and attitudes that are applied by speech and language professionals, but they will apply them to a greater or lesser extent and in a different combination. It is important to recognize that certain abilities or attributes are common to other personnel as well as speech and language clinicians, but these personnel have different roles and responsibilities and need their own special combination of what are often called competencies.

Not only do speech and language clinicians develop a core of skills, attitudes and knowledge that can be transferred to new contexts, but as they concentrate on a special field, further knowledge and skills specific to the area are accumulated. Davies and van der Gaag (1992) and van der Gaag and Davies (1992a,b), in their studies of three groups of clinicians (one working with children, one with child and adult learning difficulties, and one with the elderly/acquired neurological disorders), show that some knowledge, attitudes and skills are common to all speech and language clinicians, and some are more specific to a particular group of specialist speech and language clinicians. In both pre- and post-qualification professional development, you will acquire knowledge, attitudes and skills that are specific to specialist areas of work, for example voice, hearing impairment, learning disability, head injury or augmentative communication, as well as knowledge, attitudes and skills that are common to more than one area of work.

It is not easy to define the make-up of a speech and language clinician. In a discussion emphasizing the importance of viewing the client/customer as an individual and the ways to ensure their needs are best met by the clinician, Kineen (1994), referring to the work of Parasuraman, Zeithaml and Berry (1985), suggests a range of attributes that should be promoted. These are equally relevant to the relationship between speech and language clinicians and their clients and are defined below to stimulate an awareness of the many facets of the speech and language clinician and the quality of service that should be provided.

1. Responsiveness: a promptness and willingness to support.
2. Competence: having the required skills and knowledge.
3. Access: providing availability and ease of contact.
4. Communication: keeping the client informed in a way they understand, and listening.
5. Courtesy: politeness, respect, consideration and friendliness.
6. Security: confidential in manner and in recording and reporting.
7. Credibility: trustworthiness, honesty and keeping the best interest of the client at heart.
8. Understanding and knowing: understanding the client's needs, constantly reviewing one's own skills and attitudes, and actively evaluating intervention.
9. Tangibility: ensuring appropriate physical aspects of facilities and materials.

A primary aim of this book is to support the developing professional in the rather daunting task of acquiring the attitudes, knowledge and skills that contribute to being an effective speech and language clinician.

# Chapter 2
# Intervention

Intervention, or what in some instances can be perceived as interference, involves a decisive act to bring about change. In everyday life and beyond, intervention activities can have either positive or negative outcomes. For example:

- seeking or giving advice
- planting blame on an innocent person
- eating too much
- enabling a friend to express feelings of grief after suffering loss or injury
- introducing new tax laws.

An act of intervention can be carried out on impulse or after careful consideration of the needs of the situation and the likely end result, and either with or without prior negotiation with other parties. In all cases the initiative will be based on a theory or belief that the individual responsible has about what will be achieved by the act taken.

The intervention of the speech and language clinician is founded on professional or clinical judgements, and must be driven by a rationale or hypothesis. That is, the decision to take a particular course of action must be justified in terms of an underlying theory and knowledge of practice and the potential appropriateness of the action for the specific client. Thus there are ethical values that must be taken into account. You would neither decide against treatment nor introduce a particular type of treatment if you perceived that the outcome would be harmful or ineffective. When the speech and language clinician intervenes, it is with a view to effecting positive change, whether in the communication behaviour or attitude of the person themselves, or in altering the way others relate to the person, or in finding out more about the person to further inform subsequent intervention. The following examples illustrate something of the scope of speech and language intervention:

1. Discussing the problems of a non-communicating child with his teacher and agreeing the most appropriate way to encourage his communication.
2. Setting up a group to develop the communication skills of adults with learning disability within a social context.
3. Introducing a specific therapy approach such as:
   - Promoting Aphasic Communicative Effectiveness (PACE) (Davis and Wilcox, 1981, 1985; Carlomagno, 1994), for a person with aphasia
   - Metaphon (Dean and Howell, 1986; Dean et al., 1995), for a developmental phonological disorder
   - Personalized Fluency Control (Cooper and Cooper, 1985), for a person who stutters
   - specific relaxation (Martin, 1987), for a voice disorder.
4. Referring a child with a phonological disorder for ENT opinion and audiological assessment and the possibility of his being fitted with and trained in the use of a hearing aid to improve speech reception and processing.
5. Disseminating information packages to care assistants in nursing homes or running workshops to help them to promote an effective communication environment for the elderly people with whom they work.
6. Providing counselling opportunities for a person to reflect on the factors contributing to his or her voice disorder.

## Decision making and intervention

How do you know what intervention is appropriate, what to do and where and when to start? The answer lies in what Byng (1995) calls 'clinical intuition, or the outcome of experience'. This is not something that a clinician has been born with, but something that develops from a multitude of learning and problem-solving skills. Judgements made about the range of types of intervention to apply, their timing and ordering, and the ways in which you will use them in a particular situation will be based on your individual knowledge and experience of intervention at that time. You will be dependent on what you have read, learned, seen, discussed, adapted and tried in the past; 'Rome was not built in a day'. Even the most experienced clinician will have once lacked knowledge, practice experience and confidence, and will constantly add to, draw on, practise and appraise her current body of knowledge and skills to meet new situations. Professional development does not stop when you gain a qualification to practise, but carries on throughout your professional life. So, keep reading, watching, talking, practising and evaluating.

Speech and language clinicians constantly evaluate the effectiveness of therapy. Unfortunately, much of the reported evidence of effectiveness that is available is anecdotal rather than research-based, and there is little agreement about what aspects of intervention are effective (see Enderby and Emerson, 1995). Certainly, there is no exact way to conduct intervention for an individual. In fact, given identical information about a case, two clinicians may differ in their opinion as to what should be done. For a particular child referred with a language disorder, one clinician might, with justifiable reasons, say that intervention should consist solely of parental discussion and guidance. A second clinician might, with equal theoretical argument, say that intervention should concentrate on involving the child in a controlled learning environment with the clinician.

Intervention is to some extent a matter of what, among all the possible means available to her, works for the clinician. You should also be aware that fashions in intervention and therapies are always evolving. A speech and language clinician may chose an intervention approach or method that is currently in vogue, or alternatively one that is tried and tested but which may even be regarded by many clinicians as outmoded. Either intervention, however, may be effective if the clinician is committed to the approach, and has a sound understanding of the theoretical underpinnings and of its relevance to the desired outcomes of the case presented. To provide the most effective intervention it is important to keep abreast of new ideas, assess their value and assimilate new learning together with careful reflection on your prior knowledge and experience.

Most important, the form that the intervention takes must be negotiated with the client and often several other people who are concerned with his or her care. Both the intervention and the anticipated end result must, first and foremost, be acceptable to the client and also, as far as possible, meet the objectives of other parties, including significant family members, friends and carers, and other key professionals.

Intervention decisions can only be made according to the knowledge you have of the client, and hence their needs, at a particular point in time. The process of continuous assessment and evaluation, the assimilation of new knowledge about the client and their world, and your perceived and objective awareness of change in the client will lead you to modify your intervention decisions over time. The following examples illustrate this:

- At an initial meeting you may choose to offer rather general information to the client but at subsequent meetings, as you know more and the client can cope with more details, you are likely to gradually and selectively provide more specific advice.
- At an early session you might test out the likelihood of one or other of two therapy approaches being more successful, prior to the introduction in future sessions of a full programme of the one that is found to be more suitable.
- You might incorporate a small child into a group to develop listening, attention and general communication skills in readiness for individual therapy at a later date, which concentrates on specific aspects of his language problem.

- As you observe deterioration in a progressive disorder in a person who you have been helping to maintain some speech intelligibility, the focus of your work may be redirected on to facilitating swallowing control and the introduction of communication systems apart from speech.

Even within a single interaction with a client, you can alter your tack as new evidence and behaviours emerge. Thus, you might abandon a planned activity to encourage spoken language because the client expresses an immediate need and preference that day for guidance to improve their writing to fill in forms, or discloses concerns relating to the communication problem that need addressing through counselling. In this way, intervention and the range of strategies introduced, are tailor-made and flexibly applied in response to the shifting needs of the individual client.

Although intervention decisions are founded on your own knowledge, experience and beliefs, and as discussed above, on the needs and wishes of the persons concerned, other vital influencing factors must not be ignored. In particular, as discussed in Chapter 1, you will need to consider the extent and quality of resources available and ensure that the provision offered is equitable, that is, it takes full account of the needs of all potential clients. Numerous questions have to be answered to guide your decisions. Does your service have the staff to enable you to offer individual intensive treatment over several weeks? Do you have the appropriate specialist skills in dysphagia, child language or bilingual language that are required? Do you have the right space for a group to meet? Do the costs and benefits of domiciliary visits outweigh those of clinic-based treatment? Is it ethical to introduce a client to a computer-assisted system of communication if there is not one available for home use? Should you spend several hours in the working week with one client when there are others receiving less of your attention or still waiting to be seen for an initial appointment? In conclusion, what you would like to offer and what you are able to offer are often in conflict, and decisions may have to be tinged with compromise.

## Intervention and change

Intervention is the mechanism by which change takes place. To understand the relationship between intervention and change, it is important to appreciate that any response to intervention is dependent on the person's readiness to change, the progress they have already made in achieving change, and on whether the intervention strategy or therapy you have selected is appropriate to facilitate the intended change. You will find that different therapies are introduced according to the stage of change that has been reached, as well as a recognition of the specific subsequent changes that you perceive are needed.

The starting point for change is an agreement between the client and clinician that something needs to alter. Knowing the change(s) that you wish to bring about, the individual circumstances and the client's current level of readiness to change, you will draw on the many possible approaches that could be used and select the intervention strategies that best fit. Following this pattern, the comprehensive model of change described by Prochaska and DiClemente (1986) stresses that change involves more than a response to intervention applied at one point in time. It depends on the readiness of the client to respond over time within a cycle of stages of change – from 'pre-contemplation' to 'contemplation', then 'action' and finally 'maintenance'. The client may not move from one stage in this cycle to the next in an orderly fashion, but may stick at the initial stage and not respond to intervention or may move back and forth to different stages. Further, the stages can be integrated. For example specific treatment (the action stage) is often introduced while the person is also being given time to reflect or to contemplate on a range of aspects of their therapy programme (the contemplation stage).

The following definitions and case examples illustrate the components of this model of a cycle of change:

### Pre-contemplation

At this stage the client will not have acknowledged that a disorder exists, or that change is possible, and so will not have begun to explore his or her condition.

- In a young girl with a language delay referred by a health visitor, this stage may be represented by the mother. The mother may not have recognized that the child is having difficulties, may not have discussed her language behaviours even with those close to her, and not sought information to learn more about language development and how to help her daughter.
- A woman who self-refers because she is receiving constant comments about her voice and is being asked if she has a sore throat may not have faced up to the reality of the problem, nor the possibility that change could be achieved.

### Contemplation

At this stage the client will appreciate that a problem exists and will begin to explore the implications of change and the extent of change, if any, that they wish to make, as well as the methods for change that are available.

- A young man who stutters may be ready to re-evaluate his feelings about his speech and associated behaviours, and about his own identity, and to weigh up whether a proposed change is in his interest.

- A gentleman without voice, following laryngectomy, may be facing up to a future without conventional speech and considering the options available – oesophageal voice, surgical prosthetic speech rehabilitation or artificial larynges – and the effects of these on his self-image and his communication needs.

## Action

At this stage, the client will have negotiated a course of change with the clinician, and strategies will be introduced to effect this change. Also during this stage the client should become empowered as changes in behaviour or attitude are shaped.

- A boy with a phonological disorder may be provided with intervention involving listening to sound and word contrasts, and receiving rewards for correct recognition. At the same time the clinician may be providing positive reinforcement when he spontaneously produces correct sounds in conversation, as well as guiding the parents to extend this practice to the home environment. Meanwhile, the child's learning and success during this stage help him to learn that he has the power to manage change.
- A girl who is speechless may be systematically taught to use an electronic communicator, learning the meaning and location of symbols, and the means to select symbols to convey messages. Eventually, with appropriate support and encouragement, the child may begin to utilize the device creatively to send spontaneous messages, thus relinquishing their dependence on the clinician.

## Maintenance

At this stage change will have been demonstrated, but support is needed for it to be fully established in the client's everyday life and to enable him or her to face novel situations and people who he or she has not previously encountered with the changed behaviours and feelings.

- A man who has aphasia and has shown change in language behaviours, developed strategies to cope with a range of communication situations and come to terms with his condition, will need continued support as he begins to return to work or engage in new social contexts. Group therapy, simulations of real-life communication exchanges and therapy sessions to discuss experiences when he first re-enters old, or encounters new, social situations might be made available. In this way, opportunities are provided for him to assess whether he is making maximal use of his coping mechanisms and to monitor his acceptance of himself, and reduce the likelihood of regression.

- A woman who has shown steady voice recovery following episodes of intermittent dysphonia may be seen again after a break of several weeks to discuss factors influencing any setbacks and whether she is satisfied with the changes made.

Following satisfactory progress of change(s) through to maintenance, the clinician can confidently terminate her involvement with the client. It is important to point out here that in practice, and for a variety of reasons, intervention can be terminated at earlier stages.

Readiness to change is not merely a matter of being provided with strategies that will promote change, but also depends on factors such as physical and cognitive development, environmental influences and experiential opportunities. The contribution of these factors informs our clinical knowledge, for example:

- that a child with phonological delay cannot be expected to acquire a more sophisticated use of speech sounds before attaining an appropriate level of physiological and cognitive maturation
- that improvement in the language use of an adult with aphasia is in large part due to the degree of neurophysiological recovery
- that the therapy response of a person with a voice disorder may be dependent on alterations in the environment, such as a reduction in exposure to noise, stress and pollution
- that a child with a language delay can only respond maximally to therapy if the environment provides the right experience and encouragement.

The speech and language clinician takes these factors into account and works with them to the best advantage for the client.

## Intervention for rehabilitation or development

You will find that the readiness to change, the motivations and the aspirations are different for each client, and in part may vary as a consequence of the nature of the disorder and whether it is developmental or acquired. In recognition of this fact, speech and language intervention is often encapsulated within either a development or, for acquired disorders, a rehabilitation framework.

### Rehabilitation

An active process which aims for a person to regain his or her former ability, or where this is not possible, to reach his or her optimum physical, mental, social and vocational capacity, and to be integrated maximally into the environment.

People who have acquired an organically or non-organically related voice disorder, dysarthria, aphasia or some other speech and language disorder such as might present in dementia, psychiatric disorder or head injury, fall into this arena. In some cases the problem may be degenerative and follow a progressive course of deterioration.

Unless cognitive deficits have affected awareness and perceptions (such as in dementia, other acquired psychiatric disorders and in some people post-head injury), people with an acquired communication problem will have a clear knowledge of, and memory for, the experience of their prior speech and language function. Generally, they will want to re-attain this ability, their experience of and belief in what constitutes 'normal' communication. Unfortunately, it is common for clinicians to have to help clients come to terms with the fact that they cannot fully regain their prior communication skills.

Rehabilitation sets out to guide the client towards a new and realistic percept of normalcy, draws on a knowledge of the client's communication status and a range of other areas at the time of the onset of the disorder, and supports the client, through direct and indirect intervention, to attain the best possible outcome. In people with progressive disorders, the goals of rehabilitation will be similarly concerned with making positive change, but will at the same time have to pay particular attention to maintaining change, and will be altered to accommodate the changes that result from the deterioration in the condition.

## Development

> The lifelong, continuing and chronologically related process of physical, perceptual, cognitive, personality and social change. Intervention actively aims for the person to enhance and maximally attain his or her potential for development.

Communication disorders in children, whether congenital or acquired in childhood, e.g. developmental dysarthria, developmental language disorder, childhood non-fluency and childhood voice disorders, immediately spring to mind as requiring intervention that addresses development. Additionally, adults with learning difficulties or who stutter are often viewed as best served within the sphere of developmental approaches.

Although the parents of children with developmental disorders, and the child in cases where the disorder has been acquired later in childhood, will have some experience and percept of normal development, the client will not have a knowledge of communication functioning other than that which they have already achieved. The motivation of the client may be, for example, to enjoy the immediate experience of intervention, to minimize the distress caused to him or her by others, or to help him or her to achieve what peers are achieving. Except perhaps in the case of acquired childhood disorders, and these are not very common, children will not be striving to revisit a previous level of achievement in the continuum of development. Intervention will consider the stage of development already achieved and the future stages that the person should be able to experience, and how to encourage the person to progress.

In conclusion, among the many factors that influence intervention decisions there are certain differences in acquired and developmental disorders, in particular related to experience, potential, motivation and expectations. Once again, you will have to draw on a comprehensive knowledge of intervention theory and approaches and apply the strategies that best meet the client's requirements.

# Models of Intervention

The importance of providing intervention that is varied and flexible enough to meet the needs of the individual client has already been highlighted. Not surprisingly, there is a wealth of approaches that the speech and language clinician can draw on and apply in diverse ways when responding to the wide-ranging and ever-changing needs of the client within an individual client-centred holistic management programme. Before looking in more detail at the types of approach that you might use, more should be said about the holistic aspect of intervention. Two frameworks of assessment and intervention are discussed which illustrate the importance of incorporating the client, other people and the environment, and a range of different types and methods of intervention in the management programme. These are the environmental systems intervention approach (Lubinski, 1994) and the impairment, disability and handicap framework (WHO, 1980).

### Systems or environmental systems model of intervention

This model of intervention is based on systems theory. It can be applied to any person, since everyone is part of a system.

A system comprises a network of elements that simultaneously interact in a variety of ways, e.g. central heating, vascular circulation, work organizations and living things. Both work organizations and living things clearly demonstrate the properties of what are called 'open systems': they interact purposively with the environment at large in order to survive, they are able to maintain their internal states (i.e. self-regulation or homeostasis) and are adaptable and flexible (Huczynski and Buchanan, 1993). In such systems any two elements that interact will produce dynamics that influence all the other elements and interactions within and outside of that system.

In a factory, the elements of the system might include the production units, the computer and information systems section, the administration department, the despatch centre, the marketing department, the sales staff, and so on, which in turn have a variety of links with external agencies. If a machine in the factory breaks down, it will not just affect the supply of completed items for the next stage in the production line. It may also necessitate reports to, and investigations by, the safety regulators, cause groups of managers to wrestle with balance sheets that reflect losses, require examination by maintenance personnel, involve planners in meetings to decide whether a replacement machine is needed, and so on, engaging numerous elements of the system. Additionally, the external environment will be drawn in, perhaps because customers complain when they fail to receive goods on time, or machinery manufacturers are approached to supply an updated machine.

Now let us look more closely at this model in terms of human systems and the individual who has a communication problem. Each individual is the core of a system and possesses his or her own set of characteristics or elements, such as educational, socioeconomic and occupational status, sex, age and race, and physical, emotional and psychological characteristics, such as blue eyes, short-sightedness, screeching laugh, outgoing personality, anxiety or creativity. Many of these characteristics shift and change to a greater or lesser degree in the course of time. Thus, if a person loses his or her sight, he or she may become more dependent on others or may adapt his or her existing interests. For example, they may start to use Braille cards to play bridge, develop new interests that are less reliant on vision, use touch and listening to orient him or herself, need more time to complete tasks, experience episodes of frustration and depression, and walk with less certainty. It is the interaction of all the characteristics that affects the way the individual looks, feels and behaves. It is also these characteristics that are central in influencing how the individual will participate as a member of the environmental system beyond.

This wider environmental system of networks of relationships with other persons and the physical world can be separated into:

- a primary system: the family and extended family (e.g. a child living with a single parent, a widow living alone, a married couple living with two children while a third child lives independently from them, two men or women living in a partnership)
- a secondary system: an extended environmental system, consisting of:
  - the places and things of the physical environment (e.g. buildings, theatres, railway stations, tin openers, scissors, telephones, computers)
  - the sociocultural environment of customs, values and standards of various groups, such as churches, schools, workplaces or groups such as walking clubs, women's organizations or therapy groups
  - the economic resources available which influence the ability to access opportunities (Lubinski, 1994).

A communication disorder, whether due to repaired cleft palate, a developmental speech disorder or an acquired aphasia, constitutes one of the elements or characteristics of the individual. It will influence the way the person looks, feels and behaves, and also how he or she functions in the environment and how the environment responds to him or her. You could illustrate this with any case you have met in the clinic. Here is just one example:

*Pete*

A 19-year-old who was unemployed, lived with his parents and three younger sisters, and enjoyed lively pub outings with a gang of friends, suddenly developed swallowing difficulties and dysarthria. He had to adopt a pattern of head tilting when drinking, and closing his jaw and holding his lips together for eating. He was anxious about the sound of his speech and irritated by having to repeat much of what he said. The only way to avoid having to repeat himself was to modify the length and complexity of what he said and he felt that this was taking away his natural flow and something of his personality. Outwardly, he did not show he minded the problem and he began to behave in outrageous ways, such as driving carelessly or playing pranks, which raised a laugh and helped him retain a place within his group of friends. His speech was most difficult to follow when there was a noisy background, such as when the television was on, in the pub, or when competing against the banter of his friends in the car. His friends did not wait while he took a turn in conversation and his family was embarrassed for him, but unsure how to help, so did everything possible to minimize what he had to say.

As already stressed, a speech and language clinician must look beyond the observed features or characteristics of the disorder. You must ensure that you provide comprehensive communication therapy and to do this, intervention has to consider three perspectives:

1. Ways to help the client adapt, emotionally as well as in functional terms, to the impact of the disorder.
2. Ways to help the family and other significant people in the client's life to cope positively and maximally develop their communicative effectiveness with the individual.
3. Ways to reduce the barriers to communication and increase the opportunities for communication for the individual in the environment at large.

The following are some examples of different types of intervention introduced to address each of these perspectives of Pete's system.

1. The client
   * dysphagia therapy – analyse the swallowing pattern in drinking and eating contexts. Encourage taking of iced water between mouthfuls. Reinforce the use of already adopted and current and new compensatory patterns

- dysarthria therapy – analyse the positive and negative factors affecting intelligibility. Concentrate on phrasing and the articulation of sounds in phrases and sentences. Encourage pauses for swallowing and taking breath, providing feedback on performance. Introduce gradually less structured contexts where the content was unfamiliar to the clinician
- support and guidance – listen to Pete's concerns. Identify his positive characteristics, share ideas about why he feels people are reacting in certain ways and search for possible alternatives and solutions
- incorporate family and friends in discussion and practice sessions with Pete and the clinician in either clinic or home settings (see point 2 below)
- liaise with the person who referred Pete, the consultant neurologist and his GP to advise them of the speech and language management and the progress made, and to learn more of the nature of the medical condition and other factors that would inform future intervention decisions.

2. The family and extended family
   - through Pete, arrange for one of his mates to come with him to a speech and language therapy clinic to talk about what is involved in communication in general. Create the opportunity for Pete and his friend to express their views on each other's behaviours and consider ways to improve their communication participation
   - arrange a visit to Pete at home following similar principles to those of the meeting(s) with his friends, but also to give explanations of the swallowing and speech problems. Guide them, through discussion and practice, to work with him, giving positive feedback on his performance, improving their participation in communication with Pete, and identify factors and opportunities that will benefit him.

3. The physical, sociocultural and economic environment
   - support Pete in introducing himself to social service and voluntary organizations to seek new openings for social and work contacts and opportunities for communication which could raise his self-esteem. Encourage him to ensure that he receives maximal financial and other support so that he can access as wide a range of opportunities as possible
   - advise Pete and his family about positive and negative environments for speech, such as switching off background sound prior to engaging in conversation and making sure that the listener is facing him to gain information from visual messages rather than relying on the auditory messages of his speech that are often unintelligible.

## Impairment, disability and handicap model of intervention

The World Health Organization (1980) put forward an international classification of the consequences of disease which is based on the value of three components: impairment, disability and handicap. As was noted in Chapter 1, for the speech and language clinician, the concept of disease includes disorders that do not have a clear relation to a medical condition. The WHO classification system acknowledges that diseases/disorders have a scope beyond their symptoms and diagnostic labels. They must also be considered in terms of how they affect the way an individual feels and functions. Although not originally proposed as a model of intervention, this classification gives a comprehensive framework to guide our intervention decisions and has been adopted as a method of predicting and evaluating the outcomes of intervention by the speech and language clinician (Enderby, 1992). There follows below a brief definition of impairment, disability and handicap with some examples of each.

## Impairment

A disturbance at an organic level. A loss or disorder of anatomical, physiological or psychological structures. It relates to symptomatic and diagnostic descriptions of disease and disorder.

For example:

- migraine
- autism
- a broken arm
- Parkinson's disease
- dementia
- phonological disorder
- dysarthria
- a pragmatic language disorder.

## Disability

The effect(s) of impairment at a personal level, manifest in difficulty in carrying out everyday activities.

For example:

- An inability, reduction or abnormality in dressing, eating, reading, writing, communicating or interaction with others.

## Handicap

The disadvantages brought about by the impairment and disabilities. It reflects the individual's response and ability to adapt to his or her surroundings, and the values of peers and society.

For example:

- lack of fulfilment of potential
- poor self-esteem
- dependence on others
- lack of confidence.

By considering the impairment, disabilities and handicaps of a communication disorder, the speech and language clinician will be drawn into designing an intervention programme that goes beyond the clinical condition to address the emotional and functional needs of the client. The following case shows how impairment, disabilities and handicaps can be manifest in a communication disorder, and how intervention is aimed at resolving all three of these perspectives of the disorder.

*Tina*

A 5-year-old with a severe phonological disorder, who was largely unintelligible to her peers, family or teachers. Her hearing, motor and cognitive development were within the normal range for her age. She lived at home with an older sister and parents, who were all very protective of her. At home and school she avoided speaking situations and presented as a shy and solitary child. She was subject to teasing by the other children in the class. The teacher was aware of Tina's potential ability in comprehension, number, drawing and copying, but due to difficulties in readily understanding what Tina was saying, avoided speech exchange with her and so did not encourage Tina to express ideas. Tina often complained of being unwell before school and her attendance and educational progress were causing increasing concern.

The three perspectives of the intervention were:

1. Intervention directed at the impairment: games to increase awareness of distinctions between widely dissimilar sounds and association with word-meaning distinctions.
2. Intervention directed at the disability: introduction of signing to accompany poorly intelligible speech.
3. Intervention directed at the handicap:
   - involvement in a group with other language-disordered children, focusing on social interactions and activities with little demand on spoken language
   - encouragement of teachers and parents to create opportunities for her to recognize her successes in non-speech activities
   - negotiation of a home programme with the family in which she could take more responsibility.

As can be seen from the above cases and discussion, intervention can be applied in infinite ways.

## Intervention approaches

The speech and language clinician will identify and describe the specific intervention strategies that have been selected for a particular client (e.g. liaison with parents; teaching specific language programmes; teaching methods to introduce a particular system of communication; reinforcing positive communication attempts; discussing coping strategies; contributing to team meetings with other professionals). At the same time, each strategy will generally be explained in broad terms that can be categorized using the following headings:

1. direct and indirect
2. individual and group
3. intensive and non-intensive.

A variety of combinations of these approaches may figure in the management of clients. One individual with a communication disorder might be engaged in individual, direct and non-intensive therapy, while another might experience group, direct and intensive therapy. Additionally, as seen in the previous discussion, a client may be involved in different combinations of types of intervention at various times over their contact with the speech and language clinician. Even within a single day, the clinician may be guiding both direct and indirect approaches in the interest of the client, while the client may be spending time in both individual and group therapy. The scope of these approaches will be made clearer from the following more detailed discussion of each term.

### Direct model of intervention

Direct intervention involves the client, or a group of clients, and the clinician in a face-to-face relationship. It does not mean that the intervention is directive or didactic. Far from this, very often the approach taken is non-directive, the clinician taking the lead from the client rather than instructing the client(s) in what they should do. For example, Allen (1992) and Hubbell (1981) both describe how the clinician responds to, rather than controls, the behaviour of language-disordered children. However, more directive approaches are also encompassed in direct intervention. The operant conditioning approaches to stuttering in young children (Onslow, 1992; Costello, 1993) and motor programming therapies for acquired speech apraxia (Wertz, La Pointe and Rosenbek, 1984; Square-Storer, 1989; Miller and Docherty, 1995) are examples of more directive methods used in direct intervention. Very often a combination of methods with varying degrees of directive, or instructive, and non-directive strategies will be incorporated.

The essential feature is that the client, or client(s), and clinician are physically together in the interaction. Additionally, parents, carers, teachers or others involved in the management programme may be present.

The following are all examples of direct intervention:

• guidance in the use of computers and assistive systems of communication
• teaching sign language
• counselling
• exercises to enhance listening and comprehension abilities
• therapy involving modelling, shaping and reinforcement to encourage greater effectiveness in the use of sounds, words, grammar or other communication behaviour, lends itself to direct methods of intervention.

Even when this face-to-face mode of intervention figures prominently in a management programme, the speech and language clinician may be orchestrating simultaneous indirect intervention.

**Indirect model of intervention**

Indirect intervention encompasses all those aspects of intervention that happen outside the face-to-face, client or client group interaction with the clinician.

Examples of indirect intervention include:

• designing programmes which are explained to and then implemented by teachers, nursing staff, carers, volunteers, parents and other significant communication partners of a client or group of clients so that learning and change can take place in contexts where the clinician is not present
• consultation, by asking, informing, advising, conferring and reporting about a client or client group in order to contribute to the management decisions other professionals are making, to guide the speech and language management decisions of the clinician, and to seek resources for the client or client group
• consultation with relatives and other significant people in the lives of individuals with communication disorders to learn more about the background of the client, and the concerns, reactions and understandings of these people known to the client, and to give support, explanations and advice which will benefit the client
• setting up of support groups for carers and clients groups
• promoting awareness of communication disorder and the service provided by speech and language clinicians, and encouraging referral and access to the service for people with communication problems

- promoting an understanding of communication disorder, non-discrim-
  inatory attitudes and behaviours towards people with communication
  disorder, and factors which exacerbate or prevent problems associated
  with communication disorder
- initiating training for volunteers, professionals or other carers to
  improve their understanding about particular client groups, and to
  maximize the communication effectiveness of their interactions with
  the client group.

More about all these aspects of indirect intervention are covered later in
the book.

## Individual therapy model of intervention

Individual, or one-to-one therapy, is often called 'traditional therapy' and
is sometimes scorned as being unimaginative and failing to reflect the
communicative environment of the real world. However, not only is a one-
to-one interaction the most common context for language use but it is also
the most common context for language learning from the cradle onwards.
As in all intervention, if it is assessed to be the most appropriate type to
meet the needs of the client at a particular point in time, then every effort
should be made to respond to this judgement.

This type of intervention concentrates on a single client. The clinical
intervention may be direct or indirect and may involve several others with
a part to play in working with the client towards altering their communication and attitudes. Teachers, parents, carers, helpers and other professionals may be incorporated into the therapy, either actively or passively,
to observe, be consulted, advised or counselled. The client may be introduced to specific speech and language learning, and coping strategies, or
provided with opportunities to explore their communicative achievements, but always in the absence of other clients. Some of the characteristics of individual intervention are as follows:

- It provides intervention that is tailor-made for one client, and this can
  be modified solely to meet the shifting needs of that client.
- It can simulate the one-to-one communication partnerships that
  commonly occur in everyday life.
- It can be facilitative or didactic, depending on the therapy methods that
  are applied.
- It protects the client from interruption, sidetracking or inhibition by
  other clients. Maximal time is given to the interests of the client.
- Its intensity can be threatening for some clients, while other clients find
  this type of intervention significantly less threatening than a group
  context.

### Group therapy model of intervention

Group treatment is merely the treatment of more than one client in the same session (Davis and Wilcox, 1985). The purposes and methods employed can be vastly different, but an essential component is that by bringing two or more people together you have created a social unit in which the participants have a face-to-face interaction (Sears et al., 1988). The client is not confined to interactions with the clinician and any other attendant person concentrating solely on their own case, but participates in therapy related to the needs, concerns and behaviours of other clients too.

When forming a group, important decisions have to be made about its size, membership, structure and objectives. You have to remember that if the group is overlarge there could be inadequate opportunities for maximal involvement of all participants. If it is too small, some members may feel intimidated. As long as each member can achieve personal objectives within the group experience, and there are also some mutually acceptable objectives, members need not be common in terms of such things as background and type and severity of communication disorder. Thus, a communication group might consist of people with dysarthria, aphasia and mild dementia with various experiences of therapy, who have dissimilar educational, work experience, social backgrounds and interests. Remember, in social settings, people with diverse experiences and characteristics meet in groups. If your primary intention is to develop communication skills within a social context, a heterogeneous group should not be discounted.

You will know from personal experiences of being in a group of people, e.g. a social club, committee, colleagues, family or children at play, that individuals take on particular roles, whether by formal or informal means, and relate to each other in different ways. Not surprisingly, when participants either join or leave the group there are shifts of roles and behaviours, that is, the dynamics of the group, and even the sense of direction for the group, change. In recognition of these features of group interaction, the speech and language clinician will make a decision as to whether an 'open' or 'closed' group is appropriate to achieve the objectives set. An open group tends to have greater flexibility and formality and fewer clear definitions of structure and objectives than a closed group.

An example of an open group would be a support group for people with aphasia, where newcomers are welcome and existing members attend with or without carers, if and when they choose, the purpose being to practise communication skills, gain confidence through experimentation and share experiences with others in a safe environment that at the same time simulates many aspects of the real world.

An example of a closed group would be a group for teenage stutterers of similar ages run on five consecutive days, applying a programme of therapy adopting the principles of avoidance reduction therapy (Sheehan, 1975) and block modification (Van Riper, 1973) (see Lawson, Pring and Fawcus, 1993).

A large proportion of the groups formed by speech and language clinicians are both psychotherapeutic and task-oriented (Fawcus, 1992). The psychotherapeutic aspects provide opportunities to support the psychosocial needs of the participants, such as increasing confidence in communicating, sharing concerns and experiences, responding to disclosures relating to the communication difficulty, and practising speech and language skills in a more natural setting. The task-oriented aspects provide more specific opportunities to improve, for example, fluency, listening and turn-taking, articulation, grammar and the use of non-speech channels, such as drawing, gesture and pointing to convey messages.

In addition to groups incorporating the client, groups can also be formed for parents, other relatives, friends or carers. Gibbard (1994) gives an example of a parental training group that was held once a fortnight over a six-month period. Objectives were set for the parents and they were given suggestions of games and methods they could use to help their child and to help transfer the linguistic learning gained from the activities to everyday situations. The parents discussed and planned together, as well as being guided by the clinician.

It is important to acknowledge that just because people are brought together does not mean they will instantly constitute an effective group. Participants will need time to become familiar with each other and gain each other's trust, and to understand the methods and objectives of the group. The speech and language clinician has to help the group form, providing opportunities for members to learn something about each other, to appreciate the expectations of the various participants and the purpose of their meeting together, and to clarify the role the clinician will take. Whitaker (1989) describes this initial stage of the group process as formative and the subsequent stage of ongoing interaction as established. This reflects our earlier discussion of the pre-contemplative, contemplative action and maintenance cycle of change (Prochaska and DiClemente 1986).

An important aspect of groups that must not be neglected is that not only must we facilitate the group forming and achieving its purpose through the established stage, but we must also prepare the members for the final, termination, stage (Whitaker, 1989). Many groups will need easing very carefully into the break up of the support and relationships they have shared. This preparation for termination applies to both group therapy and individual therapy. For both settings we need to spend time with the client(s) reviewing what has been achieved and coming to terms with a new phase.

### Intensive and non-intensive models of intervention

Clinicians vary in their understanding of what constitutes intensive rather than non-intensive intervention. This is largely due to the individual experience of clinicians and their interpretations of the quantitative and qualitative factors that explain the terms. It is hoped that the following discussion will help formulate an appreciation of these concepts.

The simplest way to think of intensity is in terms of the amount of face-to-face contact time that is concentrated on a client within a given period of weeks or months, that is, the quantitative value. For example, an hour-long session of group or individual direct therapy each week, even running over several months, is not generally perceived to be intensive. On the other hand, a half-hour session provided several times a week for two or three weeks is likely to be referred to as intensive. In part, interpretation is based on custom and practice. Some clinicians may consider more than three sessions a week to be intensive, particularly where they commonly see clients for no more than a single session each week.

In determining whether therapy is intensive or non-intensive we must also consider the nature of the clinical contact, that is, the qualitative value. While three individual half-hour sessions of therapy across a week might be described as intensive, a two-hour group session once a week is unlikely to be considered as such, in spite of the longer time in therapy. Further, where therapy is more structured and directed, intervention is more likely to be perceived as intensive. For example, in the case of a person admitted to a ward with dysphagia, who we see briefly but daily, we are more likely to describe the intervention as intensive if the contact involves the introduction of a specific programme of dysphagia rehabilitation, rather than simply monitoring progress and readiness for more direct intervention.

As already indicated, intensive and non-intensive intervention are equated with amounts of face-to-face contact time. For every person receiving intensive or non-intensive intervention, a significant amount of time will also be spent on indirect intervention during the same period. We may make three phone calls, write a report, visit a school, attend a case conference, discuss progress and offer advice to parents outside of a weekly therapy session with a small child, but these activities would not be taken into account in determining whether intervention was intensive or non-intensive. It is also important to note that it may not be the speech and language clinician who is responsible for the delivery of intensive therapy. This would be the case where an assistant, teacher or parent is following a concentrated therapy programme under the guidance of the clinician.

The greater our experience of different types of intervention, the greater will be our appreciation of the scope of their dynamics and the possibilities for change that they offer our clients. In later chapters there is further guidance on specific aspects of intervention.

# Chapter 3
# Assessment: Process and Practice

If there is a complex thing that we do not yet understand, we can come to understand it in terms of simpler parts which we do already understand.

(Dawkins, 1986: 11)

Assessment appears to be a very complex area, but if you can take note of what Richard Dawkins says and build up a picture of the whole process bit by bit, you will find that you do understand it and are able to undertake the practice that it involves.

So, let us start by defining the words being used and considering the approaches you will be taking when assessing an individual with a speech and language disorder.

*Process* is a sequence of operations undergone to reach a goal (the abstract 'conceptualizing') and *practice* is the course of action or the performance of specific activities (the concrete 'doing'). The nature of assessment is to think and do at the same time, so the action cannot be easily extricated from the consideration, thus the two need to be considered side by side. As you can see from Figure 3.1, the whole process of assessment can be broken down into subsections and this is what you will need to do to decide what procedures are needed at what stage. But the gaining of information from clients is never complete, so the process needs to be thought of as cyclic – each new piece of knowledge feeds both forwards into the next stage of the procedure and backwards, causing potential changes to what you already know about your client.

In the profession of speech and language pathology and therapy, we tend to adhere to a scientific approach. This entails reasoning about the problem, based on both deductive and inductive thinking. *Deductive thinking* involves drawing conclusions from what you find out from the data you have in front of you. *Inductive thinking* is the generation of new hypotheses or ideas about what the problem might be, which can then be investigated. These processes lie at the heart of any competent work in the field of speech and language clinical practice. So, when presented with a client who enters therapy with a particular speech and language problem, you should:

- define the problem
- develop hypotheses
- plan your approach
- consider ways of collecting data
- decide which instruments might be necessary
- decide who is most competent to undertake a particular investigation, for example you might wish to take measurements on a laryngograph and need to request this to be done by a colleague in a hospital department that has such equipment
- collect the data
- carefully record the information from contacts with the client or others
- analyse the data
- assemble the information in an orderly fashion
- compare with norms or other criteria if appropriate
- accept or reject the original hypotheses
- generalize from data if appropriate.

Throughout this book, and particularly within this chapter, we will be asking you to think in an orderly, systematic and therefore scientific way, and to do this we shall start with a flowchart to help focus your attention on what you need to do and where you are going during the process of assessment.

## Defining assessment

A large part of your role as a speech and language clinician is the assessment of the difficulties your clients come to you with. You develop through your training the ability to perceive and observe the strengths and weaknesses of your clients' communicative systems (Wirz, 1995).

Assessment is 'to do with making a judgement about an individual in relation to a large group of people, based on the acquisition of a body of knowledge concerning that individual' (Beech, Harding and Hilton-Jones, 1993: xi). This can be done using either descriptive or prescriptive methods (Wirz, 1993). *Descriptive* assessment methods set out to describe in detail the communication behaviour of an individual as a basis for decisions about where problems lie and what might be done about them. *Prescriptive* assessment uses standards or norms as the basis for comparing one person with another. Both forms of assessment involve acquiring a body of knowledge about the particular client and using this as the basis for deciding on a particular course of action.

Before moving on to consider in detail the process defined in the flowchart, it is necessary to bear in mind the approaches you might use in assessment. Will your assessment be:

- a screen or a full assessment
- formal or informal

- norm-referenced or criterion-referenced
- standardized or non-standardized?

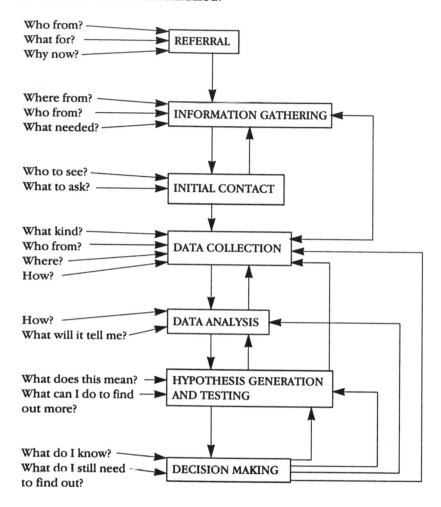

**Figure 3.1:** A flowchart of the assessment process.

*Screening vs full assessment*

Screening is a simplified procedure designed to pick out aspects of behaviour that need to be more fully investigated. In the clinical setting, you may use some play, some matching tasks, some conversation and some problem-solving games with a 4-year-old as a general screen of his performance. Based on your observations, you may then decide to go ahead with an in-depth assessment of his comprehension difficulties. Or you may use an already designed screening test such as the First (Fielder, 1993) to tap areas of difficulty soon after a client has had a stroke. Once you have a better picture of your client's levels of ability, you may then go ahead with a more comprehensive test battery.

*Formal or informal*

The division here is between the gathering of information through some pre-planned, organized or standard procedure, or through an observational approach. A test that can be bought is the most formal procedure you might use. This would give clear guidelines about administration and would very likely be both standardized and norm-referenced. An example of such a test would be the Reynell Developmental Language Scales III (Edwards et al., 1997). A pre-prepared checklist could also be considered a formal procedure. This is likely to be criterion-referenced, such as the Functional Communication Profile (Sarno, 1969). An informal approach would be individualized and would consist of observation, recording of behaviour seen and devising appropriate ways of probing more deeply into areas that you feel might be more of a problem for this client. You might start with general conversation with an adult and through this note that there seems to be some lack of intelligibility and slurring of speech. You watch the movements of the client's articulators with care, you note posture and breathing, you check for spillage during the drinking of a cup of tea. You might also ask this client to imitate certain movements of his articulators or to produce a sound such as [s] or [z] and hold it for as long as possible. Informally, you are building up a picture of this person's difficulties. As you can see, both formal and informal approaches will give valuable information and can be flexibly interwoven in the ongoing process of assessment (see Lees and Urwin (1997) for useful ideas of the formal and informal assessment of children).

*Norm-referenced or criterion-referenced*

Norm-referenced tests relate the performance of a client to peers of the same age. An example of such a test would be the Clinical Evaluation of Language Functions (CELF-R, Semel, Wiig and Secord, 1987) where each subtest can be scored in relation to the ability of children with no language difficulties. The problem of norm-referenced tests in the speech and language area is that it is often inappropriate to relate the performance of many of your clients to a norm. This is clearly argued by Dockerill and Henry (1993) in relation to adults and children with learning difficulties.

Criterion-referenced assessments give a picture of whether an individual does or doesn't have a particular skill. A carefully designed scale of this kind is based on a step-by-step breakdown of the behaviours needed for a specified skill. For example, the Wessex-revised Portage checklist (White and East, 1983) gives examples of the language understanding or production to be expected of the child, which can be easily scored as that behaviour is noted. A problem with this type of approach is that individuals do not all conform to a particular order of skill development, so criterion-referenced procedures cannot easily be used to define progress over time.

*Standardized or non-standardized*

Standardization can be taken to mean a formalized, structured procedure for the administration of a test and/or the carrying out of the test on a sample of people to gain an idea of the range of possible responses to the test items. The more people included in the sample used to standardize a test, the more sure you can be that the behaviours expected by the test are valid. For example, if you know the number of side-to-side movements of the tongue expected in 60 seconds is the mean of a large group of adults across a wide age range, you can feel confident that the fact that your client could do only a few movements in that time is significant (see Beech, Harding and Hilton-Jones (1993) for lists of tests and the populations on which they were standardized). A non-standardized assessment procedure is no less useful, but for different purposes. Many of the procedures clinicians use to assess phonology are non-standardized because what is being looked at is the child's unique sound system rather than speech sounds used or not used by others of this age group.

# The assessment process

Think of the process of assessment as the fitting together of a jigsaw. You need to find and fit the shapes to form a picture of the person you are to be involved with. Unlike the jigsaws you did as a child (or still do now), you do not have a photograph on the front of the box to guide you. You do, however, have the knowledge gained from the fields of linguistics, psychology, medical sciences, education and sociology. These theories and ideas can give you confidence in finding and fitting your pieces. Look back at Figure 3.1, the flowchart of the assessment process. We shall now take time to think about each level of this chart, and the processes and practices it involves.

## 1. Referral

Picture yourself in your clinical setting, having just received a letter or a phone call asking you to see a client for the first time. The thrill that you feel – part excitement, part fear – is one felt by even the most experienced clinicians, and it is what makes the work of the speech and language clinician so stimulating. Who will the client be? What problems will he or she bring? How will you go about solving them?

To refer is to hand over something (in this case information on a person) to another. This means that the responsibility for dealing quickly and appropriately with this information is also handed over. The expectation from the referring agent is that you will deal with whatever issues are needed, keep him or her informed and, once you have seen the person or people involved, pass your additional information on to the referrer. The referral may come in the form of a letter, a pre-printed form, a telephone call or a face-to-face contact. Your response must be as speedy as possible, however the information is conveyed. In many work districts, you would be expected to write a letter in response to a referral within a set time (e.g. one or two weeks).

When you receive a letter from a referring agent you may think 'Can't I refer this person on to ... who is much better able to deal with this sort of thing?' or 'Can't I discharge this person who has such a minor problem before seeing them?'

No! You have a professional responsibility to assess the situation. Also, the referral letter you have in front of you is the subjective view of the doctor, teacher, social worker, parent, client or whoever the referring agent is. However detailed the information, you still do not know what sort of problems (if any) the person who walks through your door will bring you. It is important that you formulate an objective view of what the problem is, and then you might decide that the best approach is to refer on to a specialist, either one in another field or another speech and language clinician.

### Who from?

Different employers may have different views as to who you can and can't receive referrals from. Make sure you know the guidelines for your particular place of work. Also remember that, even if there is a very open referral system, there are still professional courtesies that require you to inform others of your involvement. You will need to thank the referring agent and give an indication of when you hope to make an appointment for the client. Once you have completed your initial investigation of the problem (which may take one or several meetings with the client as well as gathering of information from other sources), you will need to send reports to relevant people (see Chapter 7 for further discussion on report writing).

### What for?

Referral letters may contain different amounts of information. Some are very detailed while others give only sketchy information about the person you are about to see. The letter may provide you with some clues as to the expectations of the person referring, as well as clues as to what might have already been said by this professional to the client. Look at the letters in Figure 3.2. What might these comments mean about the way in which the referrer views the problem? What do you think the expectations of the referring agent might be of you and your service?

### Why now?

This is a very important question to ask yourself before you see the client, and the client and/or carer when you have the initial consultation. The referral could be coming to you now because something has happened recently or the pressure to seek help may have been building for some

1. Referrals from a health visitor:
'Please see this little girl who cannot say her 's' sounds'
                    or
'Please see this bright little boy who can't yet talk'.

2. Referrals from a consultant:
'Please assess and advise Mrs B. following her stroke'
                    or
'Please could you see this very anxious lady who I saw in my clinic today and whose vocal cords are completely normal'.

3. Referral from a teacher:
'John cannot cope with his school work and is becoming a problem because of his speech'.

**Figure 3.2:** Examples of referral letters.

time. Sometimes the referral occurs because of an important event in the client's life. The factors that have instigated the referral are likely to be as much a source of concern as the speech and language difficulty itself and this is why it is so important for you to take account of them. Some of these triggers to referral may be:

- occurrence of a crisis (e.g. a stroke, an imminent laryngectomy)
- perceived interference by the problem with social or personal relationships such as might occur when a person who stutters reaches young adulthood
- pressure by others, for example by an employer who finds it difficult to understand the speech of someone who clutters
- persistence of symptoms after a personally set deadline as might occur when a parent suddenly decides that the child's speech difficulties should have improved by now
- relationship between the problem and other goals (e.g. delayed language in a family with high academic standards)
- access to health care facilities (e.g. either proximity and/or finance may have made access difficult but this has now changed).

## 2. Information gathering

Lahey (1988: 123) says that 'information should bear directly on identifying whether there is a problem, on determining the goals and procedures for intervention, or on determining progress'. So you do not seek information blindly, you have a plan of what you want to find out and why. Your plan must be constructed carefully, to ensure that nothing is missed. It is your responsibility, once the referral has arrived, to seek out information in a systematic way. A plan is a blueprint for the work to be undertaken. It will consist of aims and objectives as well as the actual procedures you will undergo to obtain the relevant details. A full discussion of the planning process can be found in Chapter 4.

The way in which you approach the sources of information – by letter, phone or face-to-face – will influence the type of information you can obtain. Correct procedures in making contact must be followed. Remember that good communication skills will be essential for the smooth running of information gathering.

### *Where from and who from?*

You will need to seek information from as many sources as possible, indirectly or directly. Indirect sources include:

- hospital notes
- clinic files
- letters from those who know this client
- school reports
- reports from social services
- care plans.

You may wish to ask for information directly, either in a face-to-face situation, via the telephone or in a written form via letters, e-mails etc. Some of the people you might contact are listed below, but there will be others who you may come across. The important thing is to be aware of the need to seek out information that is relevant from as wide a range of sources as possible. Direct sources include:

- client
- parent, spouse or other carer
- other involved people, e.g. friends, community contacts
- referral agent
- relevant consultant
- client's general practitioner
- health visitor or district nurse
- other involved speech and language therapists
- related professionals
  - physiotherapist
  - occupational therapist
  - social worker
  - clinical psychologist
  - educational psychologist
  - head teacher
  - class teacher
  - managers or staff at social services settings, e.g. nurseries, day centres, homes for the elderly etc.
  - employer.

*What is needed?*

A good way to think about all the information that may be needed is to use a model that enables you to recall what you need to find out. Many workplaces have a particular case history form that gives headings as prompts for your memory. You might decide to devise a model of your own, e.g. a flowchart or a diagram, to make sure you gather the relevant information.

The Venn diagram has been used by many authors as a useful tool for demonstrating the overlap between particular aspects of the behaviours under investigation. Lahey (1988: 18) has used a Venn diagram to help us conceptualize language as being composed of the areas of content, form and use which may be seen as discrete but which overlap and merge in a fully functioning system. Also Wall and Myers (1984) have used this diagram to identify particular areas of concern for children who stutter. Another model used in the stuttering literature is that of Rustin, Cook and Spence (1995: 38), which uses a grid-like framework for identifying areas to investigate.

Figure 3.3 suggests models you might use. You will need to bulk out these general models with more detail as indicated below. These lists are not conclusive, there will be other factors you can add as you become aware of them.

## Medical information

You may need to consider some or all of the following depending on the problem:

- general health – at present and in the past, how this affects the person and the problem
- nature of the disorder, e.g. progressive, acute onset, developmental
- neurological factors – evidence of brain damage or neurological dysfunction from the notes
- pertinent illnesses – upper respiratory problems or otitis media may have affected hearing, bronchitis may be associated with voice disorder, encephalitis may have led to memory loss, etc.
- sensory abilities – particularly hearing and vision where the problem may be one of acuity or perception or both
- motor abilities – gross or fine motor skills may be different from what might be expected
- ways in which medical problems have been dealt with:
  - surgical procedures particularly significant in cleft palate or laryngectomy, glossectomy, etc.
  - drugs, which may well have an impact on the speech and language, memory, articulation of the client (see Vogel and Carter (1995) for useful information on drugs, and speech and language behaviour)
- what is still being treated

A. A Venn diagram (after Wall and Myers, 1984: 7)

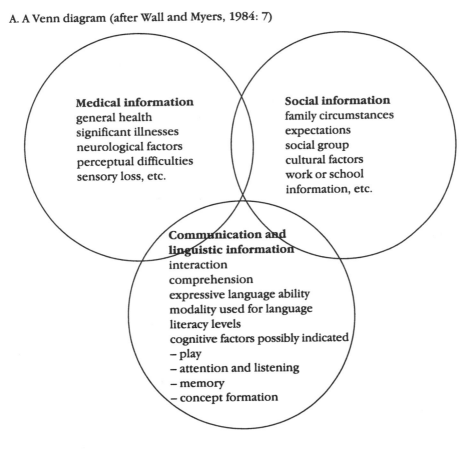

**Medical information**
general health
significant illnesses
neurological factors
perceptual difficulties
sensory loss, etc.

**Social information**
family circumstances
expectations
social group
cultural factors
work or school
information, etc.

**Communication and linguistic information**
interaction
comprehension
expressive language ability
modality used for language
literacy levels
cognitive factors possibly indicated
– play
– attention and listening
– memory
– concept formation

B. A grid model (after Rustin, Cook and Spence, 1995: 38)

| Physiological factors | Social/emotional factors |
|---|---|
| medical information<br>hearing and vision<br>motor control<br>family history<br>developmental details | awareness of problem<br>feelings about problem<br>relationships<br>emotional stability<br>social skills |
| **Environmental factors** | **Cognitive factors** |
| family circumstances<br>school/work information<br>pressure from others<br>demands of environment<br>reaction of others to problem | language<br>play<br>attention<br>memory<br>learning ability |

**Figure 3.3:** Information-gathering models.

- which medical professionals are involved
- family history – many speech and language conditions are either part of a genetic condition, such as FragileX syndrome, which runs in families, or have a familial tendency, such as stuttering where there is up to a 71 per cent chance that a child who stutters will have a member of the extended family who also stutters (Ambrose, Yairi and Cox, 1993)
- developmental information – the way in which the child developed over time and the speed of this in relation to expected norms is vital information. You will also be interested in the long-term developmental course of disorders such as cleft palate, stuttering, cerebral palsy, etc., as this will give you a view on positive or negative changes over time. Being alert to change over time will allow you to chart the progress of neurological disorders such as motor neurone disease or take account of the changes found in dementia.

## Creating a developmental profile

It is essential that you become competent at identifying differences from normative development in the children you see. To do this, you might make, as a clinical tool, a developmental profile in an easy-to-carry folder or on file cards. Your profile should cover a fairly wide age range, from birth to five years for all aspects, and then from five to adolescence for specific language skills (such as the ability to make inferences or tell or understand jokes), or problem solving and abstract thinking.

The following areas are suggested:

- physical growth including such things as head circumference
- reflexes
- gross motor development
- fine motor development
- perceptual abilities
- social/moral development
- cognitive development
- concept development and learning levels
- development of play
- language development.

Information is available from books, videos, developmental charts, lecture notes and experience in clinic and of children in other settings. The file will need to be added to as your own knowledge grows and you should cross-reference to make sure that you are gaining a full picture. Figure 3.4 shows examples of developmental profile entries.

To help you make use of the knowledge you are gathering, you must draw on your understanding of theory concerning the relationship between certain traumas, diseases, genetic conditions, drug doses, sensory loss, developmental delay, etc., and behaviour including language and speech (see Table 3.1).

You may wish to have your entries identified by behaviour:

> **Social behaviour 2.06 years**
>
> Very active, dislikes restraint
> Little understanding of common danger
> Very dependent on adult

> **Motor development 2.06 years**
>
> Walks upstairs and down confidently but places two feet on each step
> Runs well straight forward
> Climbs easy apparatus

Or you may take an age and identify a range of behaviours within that:

> **Age 2.06 years**
>
> Motor skills: gross motor – walking upstairs and down with ease;
> fine motor – builds tower of seven cubes using preferred hand
> Social skills: unaware of danger very dependent on adult
> Needs parent close by
> Language skills: comprehension – understands large
> vocabulary and SVO, SVA structures
> Expression – asks questions 'what?', 'where?'

**Figure 3.4:** Examples of developmental profile entries.

### Social/emotional and environmental information

There are numerous areas that can be considered under this heading. Some of the more common factors which may well have significance in helping you to understand the speech and language difficulties of your clients are:

- family circumstances – who is in the family, what are relationships like in the family, how does your client fit into the family structure, what are the support networks for the family, are there any financial or other pressures on the family, what are the language levels in the family, what expectations do they have for the child, what languages occur in the home, what language models are being given?
- social and cultural factors affecting the family and the client – what expectations are placed on the client for language performance from his or her social grouping or culture, what role does this client play in the social or cultural structures?
- work and school information – this will give clues as to educational status, interests, environmental factors (noise, pollutants), lifestyle (consistency, stressors, such as time pressure).

**Table 3.1:** Examples of the influence of medical factors

| Problem | Medical factor |
| --- | --- |
| Mrs S has a voice problem | This may be affected by her use of an inhaler |
| Jane has phonological difficulties | It appears that these are related to intermittent hearing loss during periods of otitis media |
| David has been in a road traffic accident | His inability to initiate purposive communication may be related to the brain damage he sustained. The drugs used to control the epilepsy which has since developed may also be implicated in his generally slow response to questions |
| Mr C is unable to obtain reasonable oesophageal voice | This may well be related to his long-term bronchial problems |
| John has a stutter | Developmental factors which may be significant are both emotional and learning difficulties during his school life |
| Ann has learning difficulties | Developmental information of significance is the emergence of spoken words at 10 years of age and two and three word combinations at 15 years. Was this just very slow development or were there significant factors occurring at these times? |

- awareness, self-esteem, expectations of self, and so on, will be important in understanding the client's motivation, level of anxiety or depression, etc.
- leisure and social involvement – this information will give some idea of health, friendships, sociability, group belongingness, etc.

Your client is a part of a system (Barker, 1996). His or her family forms the core of the system; society, school, friends, etc. form a second system, and the client's cultural background forms another larger system. All these systems are interconnected. The slow development, lack of development or loss of speech and language in one individual has implications for the feelings, lifestyle and methods of managing for those significant other people who are associated with the individual. You will need to understand how the family, school or social group from which your client comes, is reacting to his or her particular speech and language disorder. You must be particularly careful that you understand the expectations and norms of behaviour linked to the particular culture from which your client comes.

The wider family or social network is very important to consider. Think of yourself and of the people around you. Who do you rely on for what?

Who helps you when you are down? Who can you have a good laugh with? A person's support system is sorely tried when that person has developed a problem. Many of you will have come across a client who has had a stroke, for example, and who is now visited by very few of his or her previous friends. Your client's ability to cope with whatever has happened and to work for positive change will be related to aspects such as support, the number of losses he or she has experienced and the amount of life changes that have been brought about (see Table 3.2).

**Table 3.2:** Examples of social, emotional and environmental factors

| Problem | Social/environmental factors |
| --- | --- |
| Mr B has poor speech intelligibility and is unable to write as a result of his Parkinson's disease | Mr B has always been in charge of the family finances and his inability to communicate with his bank is causing both him and Mrs B a great deal of unhappiness at present |
| Arfan has a developmental language problem | At 4 years of age Arfan is in a nursery setting where English is spoken. At home his family speak Gujerati. Having two languages is putting additional strain on Arfan's immature language skills |
| Joan has a voice disorder | Joan works as a typist/secretary in an open plan office. She is often talking on the phone above the noise of machines and people. This may be a factor in the abuse of her voice |
| Mrs C has dysarthria | Mrs C has no immediate family. A niece visits her and does her shopping weekly. You feel that Mrs C's dysarthria will improve with practice but she speaks to very few people from week to week. The majority of her speaking is done when she comes to see you |

## Communication and language information

Your main aim in the assessment process is to gather relevant information about the ability of your client to use language as a means of communicating with others. Some clients you may see, such as young children or people with severe learning difficulties, may be pre-linguistic, that is they will not have developed a code for conveying their messages. However, they will all be communicating in some way or form and it is your job to identify how this communication is taking place.

Speech and language clinicians are always interested in language as a two-way system. In a communication exchange both people will play the role of the giver and receiver of information. It is vital therefore for an individual to be competent at:

• receiving the message via the senses

- interpreting the message through the cognitive processes of decoding and making sense of the information
- planning the response through the cognitive processes of encoding and organizing the message in preparation for producing it
- producing the message via the motor system.

(See Crystal and Varley (1993) for a fuller discussion of the communication chain.)

Messages can be passed via the auditory-oral system where the information is spoken and heard, or via the visual-manual system where information is provided through the hands (a signed language). These are the main systems you might come across, but you will also deal with individuals who require the receiving and passing of messages via a tactile system.

To ensure that you do not forget to notice behaviour in certain areas of communication, you need a framework or plan for your assessment. As already mentioned, the Venn diagram provided by Lahey (1988: 18) is extremely useful. Under her headings of form, content and use you may think of the following:

- *Form* means the structure of language. An investigation of this area will involve the identification of your client's strengths and weaknesses in either understanding or producing:
  - grammatical structures, that is morphology and syntax
  - word forms, that is phonology and phonetics.
- *Content* is the 'linguistic expression of what we have in mind' (Lahey, 1988: 11). It is related to the understanding and producing of words that carry the required meaning:
  - vocabulary that is appropriate to objects, events and actions
  - the relations between objects, events and actions.
- *Use* (or pragmatics) means the way in which language is used to interact with others. This involves the understanding and manipulation of the communication between individuals such as:
  - 'norms' of communication such as turn taking, use of gesture and facial expression, use of spatial and postural adjustments for different contexts
  - supralinguistic information carried by vocal tone and intonation patterns
  - conversational patterns such as making statements, commands, requests, etc., attending to the topic under discussion, saying appropriate things in response, knowing what kind of and how much information to offer, etc.

As well as spoken or signed language ability, you will need to investigate a child's or adult's literacy levels. The known links between slow phonological development and reading and writing problems (Stackhouse and Wells, 1997), as well as the importance of understanding the possible loss of these skills following brain injury (Barry, 1991) highlight the importance of this knowledge.

As well as exploring the language system directly, you will need to look carefully at those cognitive skills which are necessary for language to develop. There is some controversy about how these skills link to language acquisition (Marschark et al., 1997), but it is clear that an understanding of the abilities of your clients in these areas will give you a better picture of the constraints under which their language systems are having to function. So you will want to assess:

* attention, which is the ability to focus on and remain focused on salient features of the situation in order for learning to take place (for a useful framework of levels of attention see Cooper, Moodley and Reynell, 1978)
* auditory and visual abilities – acuity, discrimination, memory
* short-term memory, which is the ability to retain information for long enough to allow it to make links and connections to other information stored in the brain
* concept formation, which is the learning of the way in which the world can be grouped and categorized in order for it to make sense. An understanding of how things are the same and different, how they are organized into groups, how events are sequenced in time and how things are organized in space is vital for the growth of awareness and knowledge upon which language is built
* play – in order for appropriate play to develop, all the cognitive processes above are brought together. Through observing a child's play therefore, you can gain an enormous amount of information about awareness, sociability, symbolic ability, conceptual level, etc. (see Jeffree (1996) for an outline of developmental sequences of play).

The information-gathering process may take place before, during or after you have seen the client. The chances are it will occur during all three periods and for quite a time after you have seen someone for the first session. Like all clinical processes, it is not finite – there are always new pieces of information to be discovered. It is impossible to learn everything about a person and his or her problem, but if you take a whole-person view and tap as many sources of information as possible, you will begin gradually to build up a picture of your client and his or her needs.

### 3. The initial contact

The word 'contact' rather than 'interview' has been used deliberately, as the latter presupposes a formal, fact-gathering process, which may not be the best way forward for the person you are dealing with. 'Contact' suggests a more open-ended coming together which may not be directly face to face, but could be observation from a distance, information gathering on the phone or informal, unstructured meetings, as well as the more commonly expected question and answer format.

The initial contact is where you are going to gather much, but not all, of the information you have just considered. Before you meet your client for the first time you must consider your moral and ethical duty as a professional. *Communicating Quality 2* (Royal College of Speech and Language Therapists, 1996: 18) comments:

> Speech and language therapists should: respect the legal, social and moral norms of the society in which they work ... refrain from discrimination on the basis of race, religion, gender or any other considerations ... respect the needs and opinions of the clients to whom a duty of care is owed.

It is also important that you think carefully about the concept of *confidentiality*:

> Speech and language therapists must maintain professional confidentiality with regard to their clients, and must refrain from disclosing information about a client which has been learned directly or indirectly in a professional capacity ... where information is shared with professional colleagues or any other person it is the speech and language therapist's responsibility to ensure that such people appreciate that the information is being imparted in strict professional confidence. (College of Speech and Language Therapists, 1991: 18)

Some points to consider before you make the initial contact are:

- How will you make contact?
- In what context will the information be gathered?
- Who will you speak to?
- How much time will you have?
- What will be your aims and objectives for this contact?
- Based on these, what information will it be necessary to know?
- What will be your client's expectations and perceptions of the problem?

*How will you make contact?*

The way in which clients are contacted will possibly be influenced by your work setting, your time and your own style of approach. If this is an inpatient contact, you might phone the ward to make arrangements to come and see the client. The ward staff will then be responsible for telling the client you are coming. In an outpatient department or a community clinic there may be specific procedures, such as a standard letter or card that the department you are working in sends to the prospective client. This may give some information about the appointment and what might be expected on arrival at the speech and language clinic. If the client has been seen before, you might choose to make contact by phone or a more personal letter. Remember that the way in which the client has been contacted can have an effect on his or her feelings about the meeting with you.

*The context of the contact and who you will talk to*

There are many situations in which you may see the client and/or carer(s). Some of these are ideal, well-planned and well-prepared settings, others may be awkward and uncomfortable and the space, noise levels, availability of equipment and so on may be outside your control.

Your client may be seen:

- in bed or in a side room on a hospital ward
- in a community or other 'clinical' space
- at home
- in a day care setting
- in a school
- in a large and airy room
- in a small and dismal space
- on his or her own
- with one other person
- with the whole family
- in almost any other setting you can think of.

Wherever the face-to-face contact is, you must be aware of the effect that this environment is likely to have on the comfort or discomfort of the people involved – including yourself. The nature of the information you gather will also be influenced by the setting. In a very public space it would be inappropriate to talk about overly personal issues. Discussing language problems with your client or conducting tests where he or she may fail in some areas will need a quiet and confidential setting. A large room is necessary if a whole family is to be seen. The availability of toys and space is essential to encourage a child's play.

*Aims and objectives*

You do not need to know your client in order to establish aims and objectives. The very limited information you may have on your referral letter will be enough to give you a starting point for writing a plan for your initial contact.

Your *aims* or general intentions will be to gather information and to form some opinion of what the particular issues are, both from the client's and from the carers' viewpoints, as well as from your own. Breakwell (1990: 1) points out that an effective interaction 'helps you see what is happening from the other's point of view as well as your own. This helps you predict what might happen next'.

The areas you hope to explore might be some or all of the following:

- The person: age, appearance, mobility, interests, attitudes, feelings, expectations, level of functioning, etc.

- The context: school, home, work, neighbourhood, culture, etc.
- The family: family members, family structure, support, relationships between family members, etc.
- The problem: is there a problem, who is most concerned, duration and course of the problem, help previously sought, others involved in problem, effects on life of those involved. (After Priestley and McGuire, 1983)

You need to consider the *objectives* of your interview from the point of view of the client. At the end of this session what will the client have done? You hope the client will have understood why he or she was here to see you and that he or she was able to talk to you openly and felt at ease in doing so. You hope the client will have offered useful information in the areas you feel need exploring and demonstrated skills, knowledge and attitudes that will help you begin to understand his or her problem.

You will also need to consider before you see the client what *procedures* you expect to undertake in order to meet your own aims and objectives, and what activities or *methods* will be used. All of these will be contained in your initial plan (see Figure 3.5).

*Moving through the session*

Openings

The first hurdle to cross is that of names – will you use first names or surnames? You must be sensitive to forms of address that are appropriate for the ages or cultural backgrounds of the people you are seeing.

Once you have managed to establish names, you may wish to put the person at ease by asking some general questions, for example about the journey, the manner of arrival, the weather, etc. This should be carefully timed and not too long (although you may find this a very useful way of making your first informal assessment of the client's speech and language abilities).

Following the introductions, you should explain to the client and/or the carers what you have planned for the session and what they may expect from this initial contact. Most people will come not knowing what to expect but having some hopes and fears of their own. Giving an outline of what will occur removes the anxiety of the unknown and begins the process of rapport building which is so vital for this and subsequent contacts.

Asking questions

It is important to understand the power of questions either to encourage free and in-depth discussion, or alternatively to stop the flow of an interaction and to reduce responses to their most minimal. Hargie, Saunders and

You have been asked to see John who is 2 years and 10 months old and who has been described by his doctor as being uncommunicative. You will be seeing John and his mother in your community clinic where you have the available space and equipment that is likely to be appropriate for a child of this age. You write the following aims and objectives.

**Aims**
1. To obtain information on John's development from his mother.
2. To assess John's level of play.
3. To identify John's method of communication both with his mother and with the clinician.
4. To get an impression of John's level of language comprehension.

**Objectives**
1. That John will have been at ease in this strange setting.
2. That John's mother will have given information about his development and felt able to express her concerns about him and his speech.
3. That John will have completed a test of his play abilities as well as played with a range of toys (a) with his mother, (b) on his own, and (c) with the clinician.
4. That John will have responded to direct requests for objects or actions from (a) his mother and (b) the clinician.

**Procedures**
1. Observe communication between John and his mother while they engage in play using general play equipment.
2. Note John's ability to continue playing when his mother is engaged in discussion.
3. Become involved in play with John and suggest sorting and matching.
4. Give John specific directions during play.
5. If appropriate use more formal assessment approach.

**Methods**
1. Set out garage and cars, farm and farmhouse, building blocks and bag of well-known objects (have some pictures available that match these objects).
2. Use Symbolic Play Test to formally assess play skills if appropriate.
3. Use Derbyshire Language Scheme for comprehension probing or you may need to adapt questions to fit the game being played.
4. Use developmental chart for planning questions about John's development.
5. Seek permission to tape record and video record for data analysis.

**Figure 3.5:** Example of a plan for an initial contact.

Dickson (1994) suggest that questioning is one of the most important skills in social interaction. The nature and functions of questions should be further explored through their book. The important thing to remember in this initial contact is that open and closed questions elicit different responses (Figure 3.6).

*Closed questions* are less threatening to the client and to you as they give you the control over the interaction. They are good for starting off the

---

The clinician is talking to John's mother about his development and home situation.

| Closed questions | Response |
| --- | --- |
| How old is John? | He's nearly 3 |
| And has he got any brothers or sisters? | Yes, a sister |
| Oh, how old is his sister? | She's 18 months |
| And do they play together well? | Yes |

| Open questions | Response |
| --- | --- |
| Tell me some of the things John likes to do at home | Well he plays with his sister. They like to chase around the house now that she can walk |
| So would you say John is an active child? | Oh very much so. And careless. He is always knocking his little sister over. I have to watch them all the time |

---

**Figure 3.6:** Examples of open and closed questions.

session, particularly if the client is a bit unsure and they elicit useful factual information, such as age, address, medical condition, schooling, etc. *Open questions* give the client control over what to say. They allow the client to offer extended information, as well as thoughts and feelings about a situation. But this does mean that you have less control of where the questioning might lead. To use open questions competently requires a good degree of skill in reflecting, paraphrasing, clarifying and summarizing, which you will gain through courses and reading in the area of the development of counselling skills.

The skill in initial sessions is knowing when to move from one topic to another and how to lead the interaction so that the information you are seeking is tapped. You will have some time restraints and you will need to feel you know the client and his or her situation well enough to make a decision on where to go next. It could be that the client or carer is talking at length about an issue that concerns them. You may realize that this needs to be dealt with but that this initial session is possibly not the appropriate place to do so. How will you express this? How will you acknowledge the need to discuss it but at the same time encourage movement to other necessary topics? You may become aware that this is a problem that is outside your professional competence, so you will need to suggest it is discussed elsewhere. How will you phrase this comment? This is where skills learned from books on counselling (e.g. Dalton 1994; Egan 1994; Street 1994) and in experiential workshops and courses can be used.

Closing the session

Closing the session involves:

* stopping the flow of what is happening
* summarizing what has been done

- inviting questions
- giving a clear indication of what will happen next
- leaving the client/carers feeling that you have given them quality time.

What must be avoided is abrupt 'run-out-of-time' endings with clients bustled out through the door not knowing what they have accomplished and what will now occur.

Endings are difficult times for inexperienced clinicians. The pressure of having to say what will happen next is great and many clients may expect instant answers to their problems. The importance of setting the scene at the opening of the session now becomes clear. If you have carefully explained that you will gather information and make informal assessments of what the problems are, and involve the client and carer in what will happen next, it will be easier to share your findings with them and negotiate possibilities for future action.

Your options are:

- to offer further assessment
- to offer some ongoing intervention, with the client, the carer or both, or via a programme planned with the school or other professionals
- to offer a self-help programme for which the client and/or carer is fully responsible
- to offer a review following a period of time in which further information can be gathered or development can take place
- to offer a referral on to another, more appropriate, professional
- to offer support via a self-help group
- to offer no further contact.

Any of these may be acceptable to the client if they are explored with him or her and with any other relevant people, and if adequate and careful explanations are given for the decision.

The initial contact is now over. You will realize that this first meeting will have been crucial in the formation of a relationship with this client and his or her family or carers. The client will also have been forming an opinion of you while you have been making your assessment of his or her language.

You may be feeling that this session did not go as well as planned. Certain areas of difficulty may not have been assessed, questions may not have been asked, the words used to express some ideas may have been inappropriate. You may be left feeling that you still don't really understand what the problem is. Reflection and evaluation of this nature are vital skills that will encourage your development as a clinician. If you do not evaluate what you have done, what was adequate and what not, then you will be unable to plan adequately for future meetings. Remember that self-awareness is often painful. However, if you try to maintain a genuine interest in the people you see, listen empathically and attentively, trying to see what it feels like from the client's perspective, and have a warm non-judgemental attitude to your clients, this can compensate for omissions and mistakes made during the session. There will be ongoing meetings with many clients and, as with any relationship, trust and understanding will develop over time. As has already been stressed, assessment is a continuing process, so any information you feel you have missed can be collected later, and new, previously unconsidered information will emerge. The process of assessment is challenging, but it is also one of the most interesting and stimulating activities in the speech and language therapy profession.

## 4. Data collection

*What do we mean by the word 'data'?*

Data are a group of known or ascertained facts from which conclusions are drawn and on which discussions are based. During the initial meeting and all subsequent sessions, you will be interested in gathering and recording data related to the behaviour of your clients and others. Data collection is more complex than you might think and it is important to understand the possibilities and pitfalls of this task. (See Crystal and Varley 1993; Ingram 1989; Lahey 1988; Miller 1981 among others for useful discussion of data collection.)

### Clinical bias

Remember as you start to gather your data that you may be unwittingly biasing the collection process by:

- your own age, sex and race
- your personality, e.g. anxiety, authoritarianism, etc.
- conducting the session at a particular time of day, in a particular setting, etc.
- unknowingly modelling the behaviours you expect from your client
- expectation of certain outcomes from your client and consequently asking questions that will bias the answer, for example 'Do you read to your child?', where the expectation is that the parent should do so and he or she will give the answer 'Yes' to please you.

In some instances you can do very little to alter the possible biases, for example if a client decides not to tell you certain things because they think you are too young. However, you can be careful about timing the data collection, managing your own anxiety, asking questions objectively, etc.

## Initial considerations

You need to consider:

- what behaviours you wish to investigate
- where you wish to investigate them
- how you will investigate them
- how you will record your information.

### *What to investigate*

We have already covered the general areas and sources of information in our consideration of what to assess. When you are with a client, you will probably want to take special note of those aspects of behaviour that contribute to the possible speech and language disorder. So you may be gathering data on:

- communication
  - interaction
  - early communicative intentions
  - social skills
- linguistic characteristics, both comprehension and expression of:
  - syntax
  - morphology
  - phonology
  - semantics
  - pragmatics
- cognition
  - play
  - concept development
  - memory
  - attention
  - reasoning
- general development of communication and language skills.

### *Where to investigate*

The environment plays an important part in influencing people's behaviour. Any setting that makes the client feel uncomfortable will alter the amount or type of that behaviour. A child who is relaxed and playing happily in a known and comfortable space is more likely to be talkative and spontaneous than one in a new and unknown room. Visual or auditory distractions can create a less than ideal environment for the collection of speech data.

Influences on the context

The purpose of your data collection and the nature of the data to be collected may influence the context. For example, if you wish to use instrumentation such as a laryngograph, the client will have to come to the equipment. This may be an alien environment and you will need to work extra hard to help your client feel as comfortable as possible. If you are doing a screening assessment, the nursery setting might be the ideal place to watch a child interacting and playing and note down a few examples of his or her spontaneous speech as well as noticing what he or she seems to understand of the language used. If, however, you need to decide the level of this child's comprehension or the nature of his or her phonological difficulty, you will have to structure the setting and the input in order to assess the specified area.

*How to investigate*

The way in which you gather data will vary depending on whether you are doing a formal or an informal assessment. Many formal assessment procedures will provide you with information on how to gather and analyse data. So in this section we will focus on more informal, observational procedures. We believe that you will need to gather information informally as a basis for making hypotheses about the nature of the problem, and you might then use the more formal tests to follow up on these initial possibilities. You will need to understand your client's strengths and weaknesses in both language comprehension and expression. Look out for books that give ideas on assessing particular areas of the linguistic system, such as that by McDaniel, McKee and Smith Cairns (1996) on assessing children's syntax or Harley's (1995) book on the psychology of language, which has an excellent chapter on comprehension.

*(a) Expressive language*

What constitutes a representative language sample?

1. *Length* The sample must be long enough to give a picture of the type of words a client uses, the way in which he or she structures sentences and the way in which words are pronounced. Because people may produce words differently on different occasions, and may limit their topics to those that they feel competent to manage, the larger the sample the better. But time is a factor that prevents you from obtaining ideal data, so you may adopt a more realistic target of around 200 utterances or about 30 minutes of conversation (Miller, 1981; Crystal, Fletcher and Garman, 1989). At times, it may be appropriate to have a sample of single word utterances, which may be collected in a phonological or articulatory assessment. It is also important to have a sample of connected speech where you can

observe the way in which particular combinations of words affect the client's ability to sequence and articulate the sounds of speech. Connected speech samples are essential to make some analysis of your client's grammatical abilities.

As well as obtaining a sample of the form of your client's utterances, it is necessary to have data which can allow for the analysis of some of the pragmatic aspects of language. You will therefore need to record both the client and yourself or another conversational partner to analyse features of the discourse.

*2. Elicited vs spontaneous* Different samples will be gathered from these two approaches so it is best to consider using both. Elicited language can be unrepresentative, can lead to single word utterances and can fail to capture words the client uses regularly. Spontaneous samples can be difficult to gather and can be limited in the number or type of utterances. Conversely, spontaneous samples can give a good indication of the child's or adult's ability in connected utterances, while elicited samples can focus on those aspects of language that are less likely to occur in a fairly short spontaneous sample.

### Ways of encouraging speech

Eliciting

- Demand: 'What's this?'
- Encourage: 'Oh, here is a ...'.
- Sentence completion: 'The girl is eating the ...'.
- Imitation: 'This is an apple. It's an ...?'
- Model offered: 'This is a girl, this is an apple. The girl is eating the ...?'
- Forced alternative: 'Is it an apple or a carrot?'
- Recall: 'Now you tell me about it'.

Conversation

A general conversation is an ideal way of obtaining data that is naturalistic and it can also be manipulated by the nature of the questions you ask. When engaged in conversation with your client remember the following:

- listen
- be patient – don't overpower with requests, questions, etc.
- follow the client's lead
- value the client – pay full attention to what he or she does or says
- do not play the fool – that is, don't ask questions to which you obviously know the answer
- consider the client's perspective.

Play

- say nothing
- play in parallel
- interact during play with little speech
- interact during play with speech
  (after Miller, 1981).

### (b) Collecting data on language comprehension

To gather information on how well a client is understanding the language around him or her is not easy. Children and adults are adept at taking note of all the cues in the environment and using these to make sense of what is going on even when they do not understand the language. If you consider how you cope when in a foreign country, you can see the importance of visual information, body language, vocal tone and so on in helping you to decipher the verbal message being given.

Ways of gathering information on comprehension are:

- General observation, which will involve, for example, watching the child when in the nursery: how quickly does he or she respond to directions?; how much does he or she need to observe the other children? Or watching the adult with learning difficulties with a member of the care staff: how many times is the direction repeated?; how much physical prompting is the staff member using?; etc.
- General conversation where the client's ability to follow the social language of conversation and to respond appropriately (maybe through nodding or gesture) to comments and queries such as 'How are you feeling today?' or 'It's lovely and warm outside, isn't it?', will give valuable information.
- Yes/no responses where the client's ability to understand when information is correct or incorrect and whether a positive or negative response is needed can be identified, such as 'Is that tea you've got?' (when it is coffee) or 'Is your name Tom?' (when it is Peter). Remember that for some clients, the problem may lie in their inability to generate the correct verbal or gestural response to the question, that is an expressive problem, rather than a lack of understanding of the question. For many of these people, their obvious awareness via facial expression, gesture, etc. will show that they know they have given an incorrect response. But again, there will be those who cannot convey this to you.
- Word-picture/object matching, which can be done in play or in general conversation. For example, 'Shall I give you your glasses?', 'Do you want to play with teddy?', while watching where the client looks, or more formally 'Where is the cup?', 'Where is the pen?', etc. This can be built up from single words to more complex and longer sentences (see

tests for adults and children such as Western Aphasia Battery (Kertesz, 1982) or The Derbyshire Language Scheme (Knowles and Masidlover, 1982)). Remember that for some clients, comprehension will be more difficult in isolated speech than in more natural conversational settings.

- Giving directions such as 'show me your arm', 'put the ball in the box', 'point to the object on the right of the spoon', etc. can be used to probe language comprehension. You must be careful to build up slowly to the more complex commands which might use concepts that are not understood (e.g. right vs left) or are linguistically difficult, such as embedded phrases like 'show me the man in the red hat who is walking down the road' (see comprehension tests such as the TROG (Bishop, 1989) for examples of increasingly difficult syntactic constructions).

- Asking questions such as 'what, who, where, how' which require the client to work out what is being requested through an understanding of the question form. For many clients these question forms require more linguistic processing than they can manage given their language problem.

- Checking understanding of inference by asking questions that go beyond the literal meaning apparent in the context. Questions such as 'Is Uncle Chris a man or a woman?' require the ability to attach gender to certain words. 'Was Jane late for work?', following a story where it was previously mentioned that the time was already 9.15 and Jane's boss would be furious with her, demands the ability to relate new to previous information. 'Arthur walked to the shops where he met his brother and they talked about his wife' can present an enormous amount of difficulty to a client who cannot sort out which pronoun relates to whom. Harley (1995: 216) comments that 'one of the main tools of comprehension is to sort out to what pronouns refer'.

Remember that comprehension requires intact attention, listening skills and memory and your client's inability to respond appropriately might well be as a result of a problem in one of these areas. Children or adults who lack a great deal of experience will have little world knowledge to help them work out what is being said. Their comprehension of language will thus be limited. Bilingual children whose background experience may be very different from that of their school peers may need a lot of help in developing their understanding of some English words. As a speech and language clinician it is very important for your assessment of a client's comprehension that you take into account all these factors and systematically explore all the possible reasons why he or she is having difficulties in understanding language.

### Recording of data

When you are collecting a sample of language for analysis, it is vital that you record. You may do this by writing down what you hear or see during the contact with the client or you may use video or audio recording, depending on what is available. You may fill in a pre-prepared checklist or a chart of some kind as you proceed through the session. Whatever you do, it is important that you: (a) prepare for the recording beforehand; (b) record systematically; and (c) have recording equipment that is of good quality. Remember that attentive listening and observation skills can pick up more information than the most sophisticated of recording devices. You can watch accompanying non-verbal behaviour, gain information on production via lip shapes or muscle tension, and note interactive exchanges that are too subtle for a video to detect. Your data may lend itself to either qualitative or quantitative analysis, and it is best to think beforehand about which of these might be the more appropriate. *Quantitative* data, such as timing of utterances, counting of dysfluencies, recording of pitch variations, etc., can be used to compare clients with either normative data or with their own previous performances. *Qualitative* data are necessary to give a picture of the nature of the communicative strengths and weaknesses. Each has its place, and for a full assessment, both should be used.

Transcription

Once the information has been gathered you are ready to produce a transcript as a precursor to analysis of your data. To transcribe is to write out and arrange information in full. Your transcription may be:

* orthographic, that is recorded in the accepted script of the language
* phonetic, that is using standard symbols such as those of the International Phonetic Alphabet (Ladefoged, 1982) to identify the nature of the sounds spoken
* broad or narrow phonetic script, that is either a transcription that has little detail (broad), or that which shows phonetic detail (such as aspiration, length, airstream mechanism, etc.) through the use of a wide variety of symbols and diacritics.

Orthographic transcriptions are used when the analysis is to be grammatical or conversational, while phonetic script is commonly used to identify speech characteristics. The transcript may consist of just the language gathered or the accompanying situational or behavioural information can also be recorded.

Perkins and Howard (1995) cite Kelly and Local (1984: 26) who say that '... at the beginning of work on language material we can't ... know beforehand what is going to be important'. It is always amazing that patterns that have been entirely missed during the process of face-to-face discussion and elicitation can emerge from a transcription.

A good transcription allows for evaluation of change over time. The effort spent at this point in making a good transcription is therefore important in decisions about where to go next and in identifying change. Transcriptions must be objective, recording what is heard and seen and avoiding the possibility of bias. However, you are using your own listening and observation skills as well as your ability in applying the forms of transcription, such as phonetic script, and consequently, the transcript is unlikely to be as objectively reliable as you would wish. The best way to overcome this bias is to have the data analysed by more than one person. Information that can be said to be reliable is that which is agreed by at least two, if not more, observers.

There are numerous texts that give information on how to proceed in transcription, and these should be consulted to help you produce the most valid data for analysis (see Crystal, 1982; Edwards, 1993, Grunwell, 1987; Kelly and Local, 1989, etc.). To a certain extent transcription will be directed by your general hypotheses about the problem. Whether the speech sample will be transcribed in orthographic script, in broad phonetic script or in narrow phonetic script will depend on whether a semantic/grammatical, phonological or articulatory investigation is being conducted. But you must always remember that these subsystems of language are closely connected and that a disorder in, for example, the use of syntax may be evidence of a reduced phonological ability being masked by the child choosing to use simple language forms. Remember also that a decision to use a particular form of data, e.g. single words, can bias the analysis unless it is supported by other data, e.g. connected speech.

Crystal (1982) gives an outline of the main features needed in a transcription (see Table 3.3):

1. Each sentence used by the client and by the clinician is placed on a separate line and preferably numbered.
2. A wide margin is left on the right hand side of the page in order to comment on additional necessary information, e.g. the visual referent for the language, the gestures being used alongside or instead of speech, etc.
3. Prosodic features are identified (marking of tone units; the direction of the nuclear tone; other prominent stressed syllables; and degrees of pause length) in order to understand the way in which grammar is being organized.

Reliability in transcription

The less intelligible the speech of your client, the more difficult it is to be sure that you have correctly transcribed the speech data. The only way to be sure that the phonetic transcription is accurate is by consensus – others must also transcribe aspects of the data (Shriberg and Lof, 1991). Remember that no one can get narrow phonetic transcription 'right', so there is no shame in your seeking help from others. Obviously, the most useful help could come from a clinical linguist, but other speech and language clinicians or students can help to establish the presence or absence of certain features in the speech of your client. Does this mean that if you are on your own you should not bother to make a phonetic transcription? No. Perkins and Howard (1995: 31) explain that '...the very act of transcription, regardless of how accurately one transcribes, makes the transcriber pay very close attention to the speech and language data, thus usually prompting a number of testable hypotheses about the client's abnormal communication behaviour'.

**Table 3.3:** Example of an orthographic transcription

**Example:**

| | | | |
|---|---|---|---|
| 1 | T | is that a 'red car/ | Points to the green car |
| 2 | C | no nòt/ | Shakes his head |
| 3 | T | teddy thought it was 'red/ | Jumps teddy up and down |
| 4 | C | silly teddy/ | |
| | | 'green/ | Holds car in front of teddy |

Non-verbal transcriptions

So far we have assumed that your client has some verbal behaviour to transcribe. But many clients you may see will be non-verbal. What are you to do about them? This is where video recordings can be of such benefit. Within an interaction there are numerous behaviours to be recorded on paper – eye contact, facial expression, gesture, vocalization, posture – all give indications of the communicative ability of your clients. (For an excellent example of such a transcription see Wootton 1989.)

Instrumental measurement techniques

Speech and language clinicians are trained to have highly developed perceptual skills, both auditory and visual, but there are times when an instrument is needed to give information that is simply not available to our eyes or ears. For example, a child may be making a contrast between two productions that can only be detected by noting a fine difference in voice onset time between one and the other sound, or an adult with a long-term articulatory problem may be making unusual compensatory contacts between tongue and palate. Instruments are used to give objective information on:

- articulation, that is the movement and contact of speech organs
- acoustic measures, such as frequency and intensity of a sound.

Table 3.4 gives an outline of some of the instruments that may be available to you, what they measure and when you might use them.

**Table 3.4**: Instrumental measurement in speech and language disorders

| Instrument | What measured | Why used |
|---|---|---|
| Electropalatograph | Lingual-palatal contact patterns | Visual feedback for articulatory placements |
| Nasometer | Nasal-oral airflow | Velopharyngeal competence |
| Videofluoroscope | X-ray of supralaryngeal cavities | Swallowing difficulties, velopharyngeal incompetence |
| Videostroboscope | Viewing vocal fold behaviour in real time | Detection of possible cause of voice disorder |
| Spectrograph | Patterns of air vibration caused by speech | Identification of phonetic features of speech production |
| Visispeech Speech Viewer, etc. | Edits real speech and synthesizes artificial speech | Gives visual feedback on parameters of speech production |

## 5. Data analysis and evaluation

*What is analysis?*

Analysis is the systematic examination of the information you have gathered and determination of the general nature of the behaviours you see.

Before proceeding to consider ways in which you might systematically examine the data you have gathered, you must first be alert to the possibility of bias. We have commented on bias before, but it is important enough to revisit in the light of the process of analysis that you are about to undertake. So remember you must set out to minimize bias by:

- being aware that you are subject to it
- using and keeping taped or videoed information
- sharing findings with a colleague
- standardizing your own behaviour during assessment as much as possible to avoid giving additional cues to your clients.

To make your data more manageable, to find what you are looking for more easily and to begin the process of understanding the nature of what you are seeing, it is wise to organize what you have recorded in a systematic way.

*Procedures for organising data*

A. Linear arrangement

1. *Alphabetical ordering*: this is of use when you have a number of single words that you need to be able to find easily. It may also give you clues regarding the variability or stability of production of a particular initial phoneme. A set of phonological data or single words uttered by a child in the early stages of expressive language development can initially be arranged in this way (see Table 3.5).

**Table 3.5:** Examples of alphabetical ordering of data

| Word spoken | Child's pronunciation |
|---|---|
| Adam | 'de |
| apple | ?epu |
| | |
| baby | bebe |
| bottle | bobo |
| bread | be |

2. *Chronological ordering*: for longitudinal data, for example utterances collected by a parent at home over months, play behaviour seen at nursery over a number of weeks, or changes in extent or range of movement over time in a client with Parkinson's disease, it is important and useful to present the information in a clearly dated chronology. For example:

**Child with developmental delay**

2.2.93    Picked up ball and dropped it 5 times.
4.4.93    Transferred ball from one hand to the other once.
24.6.93  Holds objects in either hand and transfers from one to the other easily.

B. Categorical arrangement

To gain information about the nature of the behaviours you have observed, you may wish to organize them in particular categories, e.g. word classes for semantic or grammatical information, semantic fields, types of play, etc. (see Table 3.6).

More complex organizations of language behaviour will be needed to identify grammatical categories or phonological processes and you are strongly advised to become competent at these. Books such as those by Crystal, Fletcher and Garman (1989), Fabb (1994) and Grunwell (1985) are highly recommended (see Figure 3.7).

**Table 3.6:** Examples of simple categorical arrangement of data

**1. Organizing words understood by a child into semantic fields (e.g. people)**

| Family | Others | Jobs | Character |
|--------|--------|------|-----------|
| Mummy | Friend | Milkman | Happy |
| Daddy | Man | Postman | Nasty |
| John | | | |

**2. Organizing words used by a child into word classes**

| Nouns | Verbs | Adjectives |
|-------|-------|------------|
| Baby | Go | Hot |
| Boy | Give | Nice |
| Biscuit | Yumyum (eat) | |
| Car | | |
| Dog | | |

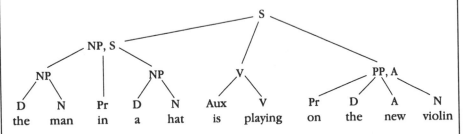

**(a) Following the LARSP (Language Assessment, Remediation and Screening Procedure; Crystal, Fletcher and Garman, 1989)**

| the | man | in | a | hat | is | playing | on | the | new | violin |
|-----|-----|-----|-----|-----|-----|---------|-----|-----|-----|--------|
| D | N | | D | N | Aux | V | Pr | D | A | N |

| NP | Pr | NP |
|----|----|----|

| NP, S | V | PP, A |
|-------|---|-------|

**(b) In the form of a tree diagram (Child Grammar, Fabb, 1994)**

```
                                    S
                   NP, S                              
           NP          NP           V            PP, A
         D   N    Pr  D   N    Aux   V      Pr   D    A    N
        the man   in  a  hat   is playing   on the  new violin
```

**(c) Two phonological processes found to be operating in a child with learning difficulties (Grunwell, 1985)**

**1. Syllable structure process: final consonant deletion**

| Target | Child's realization |
|--------|---------------------|
| /kat/ | [ka] |
| /pig/ | [pi] |
| /haus/ | [hau] |
| /bath/ | [ba] |

**2. Substitution process: stopping of fricatives**

| Target | Child's realization |
|--------|---------------------|
| /sun/ | [tu] |
| /farm/ | [ka] |
| /shoe/ | [tu] |

**Figure 3.7:** Examples of grammatical and phonological arrangements of data.

Always remember when you are analysing grammatical constructions that characteristics of spoken English may follow an unusual form, not because the client is disordered, but because he or she has another language as the mother tongue. Word order may be affected. In Bengali, for example, the basic subject-verb-object structure which we are so used to is replaced by a subject-object-verb structure, or words such as negatives will appear at the end of the sentence (see Duncan (1989) for further examples).

## C. Coding

This is simply a way of identifying when particular behaviours occur within a continuous sample. For example, when noting the occurrence of an initiation or a response within a conversation, one may simply mark an I or an R by the noticed behaviour. Or in identifying the number of repetitions or prolongations that are occurring one may mark an R or a P at the point of occurrence.

These can then be counted to arrive at a quantity of the particular behaviour and this can then be compared to what may be expected, or to some criterion previously identified (see Figure 3.8).

---

**(a) Lack of initiations in the conversation of a brain injured young adult**

| | Speaker | Utterance | Coding |
|---|---|---|---|
| 1 | Therapist | /what have you been 'doing todày/ | I |
| 2 | Paul | /I went 'out/ | R |
| 3 | Therapist | /where did you 'gò/ | I |
| 4 | Paul | /'swimming/ /yeh 'swimming/ | R |

(long pause during which therapist waits to see if Paul will add more information)

| | Speaker | Utterance | Coding |
|---|---|---|---|
| 5 | Therapist | /would you like to 'tell me something about the swìmming/ | I |
| 6 | Paul | /'no/ | R |

**(b) Identifying repetitions and prolongations in stuttered speech**

```
          R        P        P        R
   P    I I I I think I w:::::ill go to the c::::::::in e e e ema
```

---

**Figure 3.8:** Examples of coding language behaviours.

## D. Profiling

> A profile is a chart containing an organized collection of categories, which represent the structural contrasts available in a language – the various sounds, grammatical patterns, lexical items and so on. (Crystal 1982: 5)

Some examples of well-known profiles in speech and language assessment are:

1. LARSP (Crystal, Fletcher and Garman, 1989), which is presented in a single-page profile chart that contains information from the grammatical analysis of the data. Crystal stipulates that a profile should:
   - provide a comprehensive description of the client's data
   - provide an organized grading of the data
   - show the influences that operate on the client's language as he or she interacts with the interlocutor (Crystal, 1982: 4).
2. Vocal Profile Analysis Scheme (VPAS), which was developed from work by Laver in 1968 (Wirz and Beck, 1995) and provides a framework for analysis of both normal and disordered voice.
3. The Psycholinguistic profile (Stackhouse and Wells, 1997), which provides a way of considering how the speech and language problems may arise from possible breakdowns or lack of development in language input, storage or output (Stackhouse and Wells, 1997: 7). Psycholinguistic processing models such as those of Levelt (1989) enable you to visualize what might be happening when language is being decoded or encoded by the brain.

It must be remembered, however, that a profile is purely a chart and that anyone can devise a chart to provide an appropriate examination of the data that are available. Dodd (1995), for example, provides a profile to pull together a number of different aspects of the linguistic system for contrast and comparison of information. She offers a diagnostic chart that looks at articulation of phones, phonological processes and rules, severity, and causal or maintenance factors. We shall be using an approach similar to this later in the chapter as a way of comparing information from two clients.

The ability to collect and organize information in the above ways presupposes knowledge and ability in identification and description of behaviour gained through the study of linguistics, psychology, medical sciences, etc. There is no short cut to these abilities. Study and careful training of your own visual and auditory perceptual processes is the only way to achieve the necessary degree of accuracy in assessment.

### Evaluation of information

You now have in front of you a good sample of data related to the problem that your client has brought to you. You have collected and organized the data in an appropriate form so that they can be clearly seen and considered. What will you now do with the data? You need to evaluate what you have in front of you. What is the meaning of what you see and how can you arrive at useful conclusions from the information you have? Think of a jigsaw analogy – you have collected most, if not all, of the pieces, and now you are beginning to put them together in the hope that you will be able to make sense of the picture they are forming. There are several ways of doing this.

## A Counting

A useful starting point is through the simple practice of counting. Counting how many times a particular behaviour occurs can be useful information in terms of the strength of that behaviour. A child who uses 20 nouns in the course of a 15-minute interaction will be different from one who uses ten nouns, seven verbs and three adjectives, although the word count is the same. Both of these children will be very different from the child who uses only three words in the same time and this child will differ from one who uses three words but 17 communicative gestures. A profile such as LARSP uses a simple count as the way to identify how much of the sample follows a particular theme or pattern. Thus you can note how often the child uses a SVC (subject verb complement) structure versus how often he uses a SVCA (subject verb complement adverbial) as a means of assessing how complex his utterances are.

## B Communicative competence

The second and a most useful approach to evaluation of the data is to look for what the client can do well – how well can he get his message across. So, for example, an analysis of the pragmatic functions of the conversation of a client with aphasia may well show that this person is questioning, requesting, stating, negating, etc., despite few full grammatical utterances (see Table 3.7). You might also notice this client's competence in repair, turn taking, or maintaining topic. Or you may be analysing information from a video of a mother interacting with her non-verbal child. Here you see that the child and mother are sharing attention to objects and events in the environment and this allows the parent to identify what the child needs. Some useful tools for identifying pragmatic features in adults or children with language disorders are the Conversation Analysis Profile for People with Aphasia (Whitworth, Perkins and Lesser, 1997) and the Test of Pragmatic Language (Phelps-Terasaki and Phelps-Gunn, 1992).

## C Error analysis

Just counting the number of errors that a client produces is not particu-

**Table 3.7:** Communicative competence in a conversational exchange

| | | |
|---|---|---|
| T | How are you today Mr A? | |
| B | Yes, yes OK/ | Appropriate response |
| | You?/ | Socially appropriate question – follows social rules |
| T | I'm fine thanks. Tell me about your week | |
| B | Monday ... Tuesday ... out ... good/ | Gives information |
| | Um ... ted ... um ... next one... no er Wezday | Self-repair |
| | No....not good/ | Uses negation |
| T | Oh, were you ill on Wednesday? | |
| B | Say again/ | Asks for repair |
| T | Ill ... poorly | |
| B | Ah, yes ... um (points to head)/ | Continues conversation, adds information |
| T | But you're fine now? | |
| B | Yes ... thanks/ | |
| | You ... picture?/ | Initiates new topic |

So, despite grammatical difficulties, this client is competent in a conversational exchange

---

larly useful. However, an analysis of what the errors are and how they differ from the expected behaviour is very useful in planning of treatment. It is also important to consider what the error is telling you. You can gather a great deal of information about the strategies a client is using to overcome or circumvent a difficulty. Thus in a phonological analysis, by noting that a child is fronting velar plosives /k/ /g/ – [t] [d] you have a notion of a possible systematic process being used by this child. You can now go on to see whether other groups of sounds are fronted, whether fronting takes place only in certain consonant-vowel relationships and so on. An adult with learning difficulties may be unable to complete the section on the TROG which deals with passives. You may notice an obvious understanding of the concept of actor and agent and an inability to give the actor role to an inanimate object. Thus 'the man is being pushed by the car' will be perceived as 'the man is pushing the car'. Such careful consideration of the direction of errors in speech and language will form the basis of your therapy. However, you must beware of oversimplification, for example you might listen to speech samples and 'phonemicize', i.e. 'tidy up', a client's phonetic output so that it fits into your pre-arranged programme of therapy (Gardner, 1997). A narrow phonetic transcription of the speech of a client with complex difficulties may lead you to a realization that meaningful contrasts are being made in the speech system but by the use of non-English sounds (for example implosives, clicks, etc.) (Parker and Irlam, 1995).

The example in Table 3.8 shows how you can use an error analysis with a child with semantic-pragmatic difficulties to identify an awareness of the nature of the topic, even though the ability to use the correct form of language to indicate cohesion is lacking. Cohesion is the tendency for communicative partners to relate their utterances to the topic under discussion and to relate back to what has been said beforehand. A child or adult with a conversational disability will find this difficult.

**Table 3.8:** Example of a careful analysis of errors in a language sample

| 1 Teacher | /did you go 'out todày/ | |
| 2 Child | /go òut/ | Shows attending behaviour |
| 3 | /go swìmming/ | Links to reason for often leaving the school building |
| 4 Teacher | 'no/ | |
| 5 | you go swimming on tuèsday/ | |
| 6 Child | it my bìrthday/ | Following previous train of thought as had a swimming party on her birthday |

So, it becomes apparent that the child is actually attempting to participate in conversation even though these attempts appear to include errors of cohesion.

### D. Overall analysis of strengths and weaknesses

If you have done some or all of the procedures above, you will have a knowledge of how often certain behaviours occur, how close to or far away from expected behaviours these are and how useful behaviours are in enabling the individual to communicate. You can begin to list the strengths and weaknesses of this person's linguistic system as a preliminary to understanding what are the important factors in the equation which will eventually lead to decisions and priorities in management.

### Case discussion: Mrs B

Mrs B was referred by her GP. She had had a stroke nine months previously, had had some therapy in the early stages but had then been discharged. Her GP felt that she had shown some positive changes recently and that both she and her husband might benefit from therapy. You arranged to see Mrs B in the outpatient department of the local hospital. She was brought in by hospital transport, which meant that she had been collected very early from home and had been driven around for some time before you saw her. You therefore had only a short period of time with her and you formed some opinion about her difficulties.

Following this, you arranged to see Mrs B at home with her husband. In this setting, things were very different. Mrs B was much more relaxed and not tired. Her profile of strengths and weaknesses was now very different (see Table 3.9).

**Table 3.9:** Mrs B's strengths and weakesses in two different settings

**(a) In the clinic**

| Strengths | Weaknesses |
|---|---|
| Showed willingness to communicate | Tired very easily and lost attention |
| Participated in social conversation by smiling and nodding appropriately | Unable to follow specific directions to point to certain objects |
| Used spontaneous gesture to indicate place (pointing) and tiredness (closed and opened eyes) | Very limited verbal output – some jargon words only. Unable to complete any formal assessment |

**(b) In the home**

| Strengths | Weaknesses |
|---|---|
| Gave many socially appropriate responses to questions using yes and no and some social phrases | Rather distracted by noises and activity in the home |
| Named familiar items with some groping, but intelligible | Tended to try and speak rather than use gesture |
| Able to complete comprehension subtests of the WAB with 75% correct | |
| Interacted well with husband who was very supportive | Some tendency for husband to take control |

Looking at Mrs B's profile so far, you are able to see that there has been much improvement in her comprehension, based on the information in her notes from six months previously. It is obvious that when she is tired, as she was when she came to clinic, she is unable to concentrate sufficiently and so cannot respond as well as when she is relaxed and alert. However, she still has some problems controlling her attention. It appears that her speech is very limited, but she shows some positive abilities in gesture. You feel you have started building a picture of her strengths and weaknesses, which you will need to extend before you can decide whether intervention is appropriate.

### E. Collating all information gathered

Once you have a wide range of information gathered from various sources and from your own assessments, you need a way to pull it all together so that you can begin to see what is important and what is not.

A grid similar to that used by Rustin et al. (1995: 38) is one of a number of ways that can help you visualize the trends that are emerging from your data collection. What is important is to organize the information in such a way as to make your evaluative judgements and decisions follow logically from the data you have access to.

Case discussion: Mrs B continued

Following further exploration of Mrs B's difficulties through informal and formal assessment, discussion with her and with Mr B and from some liaison with the speech and language clinician who had previously seen her and with her GP, you arrive at the overall picture shown in Figure 3.9.

| | |
|---|---|
| **Medical and developmental factors**<br>Has bronchitis often in winter<br>No extension of original stroke<br>Mobility poor and no change over time<br>Some reduction in hearing since stroke | **Social/emotional factors**<br>Mrs B gets upset if she is unable to<br>achieve a task (as in the tests)<br>Mrs B very dependent on Mr B<br>Very social and socially capable, but<br>goes out very little |
| **Environmental factors**<br>Home has been adapted but she finds<br>it difficult to get out of the house<br>Husband is retired and has taken over<br>all household tasks<br>No children and limited circle of friends<br>Previously Mrs B very keen on knitting<br>but now cannot manage<br>Television often on | **Communication and language**<br>Good functional communication<br>Comprehension good until long,<br>complex directions given<br>Hearing loss makes for difficulties when<br>there is background noise<br>Limited verbal ability – only a few social<br>words intelligible – but Mrs B can<br>spontaneously write single words when<br>encouraged |

**Figure 3.9:** Overall summary of Mrs B's difficulties.

It is possible to see from this grid that Mrs B's problems are primarily those of an environmental and social nature. True, she has major expressive language difficulties, but she is able to communicate her needs well. However, there are environmental changes that would enhance her ability and wish to communicate, such as reduction in background noise (the television) and increased independence. Encouragement in the use of her strengths – her gesture and writing – could compensate for some of her verbal difficulties. You are now clearer as to the direction that intervention may take. This overall visual picture has helped you to make sense of all the data you have so far gathered.

## 6. Hypothesis generation and testing

A hypothesis is a clear statement about the relationship between two things (ideas, events, symptoms, etc.). Generating a statement of this sort helps you think about what you know and don't know about how these two factors relate and so will guide you to consider what further investigations may be necessary. The statement should be in some way testable, that is you should be able to think of a way to find out whether X really does relate to Y. Hypotheses should be made at all stages of assessment and intervention. By proceeding in this way you are deciding which pieces of jigsaw fit and which need to be discarded as you go along. It is easiest to see what is meant by a hypothesis by working through an example and showing what sort of hypotheses might be made at different stages of your assessment.

Case discussion: Lisa

Lisa is 7 years old. She was referred by her school, as she was having difficulty reading. The teacher said she had a slight speech problem but nothing they were worried about.

You have found that Lisa was known to the speech and language therapy service when she was between 3 and 4 years old. She presented with a fairly severe phonological delay, but this had remediated with therapy. At the time of her discharge she had a full phonetic inventory and the only phonological immaturities were some cluster reduction in /s/ clusters and gliding of /r/. There were no medical or developmental factors that were significant.

> **Hypothesis 1** The known relationship between phonological delay and reading difficulties suggests to you that this might be the area to investigate in detail when you see Lisa. You hypothesize that Lisa will show some metaphonological difficulties, that is, she may have difficulties understanding that words are composed of syllables and that syllables are composed of parts such as the onset (the beginning consonant) and the rhyme (the following vowel and consonants).
>
> **Hypothesis 2** However, you have no information on the rest of her language system or on her general learning ability, so these could also play a role in her reading problem. You hypothesize that Lisa will show some delay in comprehension and/or expression of grammatical or semantic aspects of her language.
>
> **Hypothesis 3** As early reading ability may be linked to exposure to books, you hypothesize that Lisa's home has few books available or that Lisa had a past history of attention difficulties and/or reduced hearing or listening ability.

The initial contact with Lisa and her mother takes place in a clinical setting and you have assembled the appropriate materials: formal tests of metaphonology (rhyming, sound and syllable awareness using the Phonological Awareness Procedure; Gorrie and Parkinson, 1995), comprehension of grammar (Test of Reception of Grammar; Bishop, 1989) and vocabulary (British Picture Vocabulary Scale; Dunn et al., 1982), as well as a range of dolls, books, paper and crayons, etc. to encourage spontaneous conversation and discussion.

Lisa's mother talks about the books in their home and Lisa's enjoyment of books and stories, and comments on the fact that Lisa insists on a story at bedtime each night. She also reports that Lisa has always loved books and has always enjoyed quiet activities such as crayoning, etc. Lisa is apparently doing well at school except for the fact that she has been unable to move beyond the first, logographic stage of reading on to a level where the relationship between graphemes and phonemes is established. So you immediately know that your third hypothesis has been refuted.

You find that Lisa is very chatty and you record her speech as she describes her home and her 2-year-old brother. You notice that Lisa still glides her /r/, as her brother's name is Robert, and that she appears to have a fast rate of speech and will occasionally delete weak syllables during stretches of speech. Formal testing on the comprehension tests, which Lisa enjoys, shows no difficulty in grammar but you feel that there appears to be some lack of vocabulary, particularly as her home is obviously a fairly verbal one. So you are forming the impression that your second hypothesis is partially but not fully refuted.

Lisa enjoys rhymes and can say a number of children's rhymes and sing some songs. However, she does find it difficult to pick out the rhyming pair from a selection of pictures. She is very good at 'I spy', showing that she recognizes the onset of words, but is very poor at noticing when the rhyme is the same (unless she can see the words such as look, book, cook). She is caught out when words rhyme but do not look the same (e.g. bought and fort). So you are fairly clear that your first hypothesis is correct and that Lisa has some difficulties at the metaphonological level which are slowing the development of her reading skills.

You are now ready to discuss with Lisa's mother and with her school the area of her difficulties and to decide whether she needs intervention from you, from the special needs department at school or from a combined programme. Further assessment based on what you have found and what all involved – Lisa, her family, the school – have identified will be needed to develop a useful programme of help for Lisa.

This is just one example of hypothesis generation and testing. This process will take place either overtly or covertly throughout your assessment of a client or clients. As you gather more information, you will feel confident to ask additional questions of your data and fill in gaps in your knowledge. You are trying to build a whole picture of the person and the situation and the relationships between these two.

You have now completed the process of data gathering, analysing and evaluating. You have tried to pull together the strands of the information, you have used models to help organize and visualize what you have seen and heard. As you have proceeded, you have used the known information to help you generate hypotheses about what might be a problem and what might need further assessment. Your next activity will be a consideration of everything that you know and from this you will need to make decisions on what you might be able to offer this client and his or her family.

## 7. Decision making: prognosis and priorities

It is always difficult for an inexperienced clinician to foresee what the outcome of a particular difficulty is likely to be. With experience, it is possible to get some idea of patterns that help in making a prognosis, but even when the features of the difficulty seem similar to those seen before, the individuality of each client and his or her circumstances demands that you be cautious in your final decision. However, you cannot avoid making some kind of prognosis even if it is very tentative. Your client will want to know if he or she can be helped and how long it might take. Your employer will want to be assured that this is the sort of problem that can be alleviated in some measure via therapy and you are not therefore wasting precious funds.

So what are the factors that can help you decide on likely outcomes and the decision to intervene or not? We will use a framework offered by Dodd (1995) to systematically consider the available information and the significance of this. We will consider factors in relation to:

- the nature of the language disorder
- severity
- age
- causal and/or maintaining factors.

### *The nature of the language disorder*

There are known characteristics associated with certain disorders that can help you decide what level of outcome is realistic. For example:

- A phonological delay affecting only one or two processes is more likely to remediate fully over time than a more pervasive disorder of the sound system.
- A chronic stutter is known to be lasting where a language delay may 'catch up' over time.
- A progressive disorder takes a certain known course, although the time span differs, while an acute acquired difficulty, as a result, say, of a traumatic brain injury, will have a less predictable outcome dependent on medical and other factors.

### *Severity*

Generally, the more severe a condition, the more difficult and long term will be its remediation. When considering severity, however, you need to ask what you mean by this. Severity must be considered in medical terms, social terms and in terms of life change, as well as in relation to the extent of the communication breakdown. For example:

- The loss of a larynx is very severe, but the likelihood of being able to communicate fully and effectively may be less affected than when the person is aphasic following a stroke.
- Communicative effectiveness would seem to be a good measure of severity, but this would not be the case in, for example, a voice disorder in a professional singer where communication would be unaffected to any major extent but livelihood would be the determining factor.
- An adult who stutters shows a high percentage of dysfluent behaviour with a number of associated movements and a high degree of tension in the musculature. He has a severe stuttering symptom. However, this person holds down a good job, has a family and many friends and has come to therapy because he is concerned about the effect his stuttering might have on his young son's speech development. So his needs for therapy would be very different from those of someone who has allowed his stutter to considerably restrict his life.

### Age

Age plays a major role in the decision equation. This may be in relation to what services are available to the client depending on his or her age, or it may be about availability or amount of input that is considered appropriate at certain ages. But remember, it is written into the code of practice that you must not discriminate on the grounds of age. If a client appears to need a particular treatment it is morally wrong to withhold it just because the client is very elderly.

Some examples of the significance of the factor of age are:

- Age of onset can give clues as to the nature of the disorder in, for example, children on the autistic spectrum or people who are dysfluent. So you will use the factor of age to help make a differential diagnosis between, for example, a stutter and normal non-fluency.
- The age at which a disorder or delay is identified and intervention is begun is very important, for example in hearing loss, stuttering, specific language impairment where it is known that early intervention can prevent some of the more pervasive aspects of the problems developing.
- Intervening before a difficulty is identified in 'at risk' children is being promoted by a number of managers and clinicians.
- Age of onset of an acquired disorder may have considerable implications both medically and socially and consequently on possible treatment outcomes. Factors such as general health, possible extension or progression of the complaint, support networks, etc., may be age-related.
- Age of the client at this particular point in time will be significant in terms of social, vocational, educational and interpersonal factors all of which may have an effect on the general motivation of the client.

- Age in relation to length of time since the onset of the condition is important, as, generally, the longer the problem has existed, the more difficult it is likely to be to change

*Causal or maintaining factors*

In many of your clients there is no clear cause of their speech or language difficulty. Even where there is an obvious medical cause, as in cancer leading to glossectomy, the environmental maintaining factors in relation to each client will make decision making different on every occasion. It is acknowledged that most developmental language problems are multi-causal, so you need to think broadly of all the possible contributors to the difficulty. Some of these factors may become the focus of your therapy, as for example when you decide to work directly with the teachers of a child with pragmatic disorder because you feel that they are unaware of the problem. Others will give some sense of the way in which you may need to offer therapy, for example you may offer short-term intensive therapy to a child with phonological delay and her parents because you are aware of the pressure of impending schooling building in the household. At times, a knowledge of the causal or maintaining factors will lead you to a decision not to intervene, for example if a client with advanced multiple sclerosis has reached a life-threatening point and his family do not wish to be 'bothered' by professionals.

Some further examples of the influence of knowledge of these factors in your decision making are given below.

Organic factors

- Structural differences, for example cleft palate, which might make remediation of phonological and articulatory problems more long term.
- Chromosomal or genetic factors, which may be associated with complex speech and language problems as in Down's syndrome, for example, where the need for some form of intervention may exist throughout the life span.
- Obvious brain damage, which will mean that complete recovery is unlikely.
- Other possible neurological function differences as suggested by attention problems, perceptual problems, auditory processing difficulties, comprehension lack, learning difficulties, etc., all of which may make language learning more difficult.
- Any sensory difficulties (e.g. hearing or vision) that are likely to affect decisions about the nature and timing of remedial help.
- History of delayed development or familial or genetic predisposition that may indicate the likelihood of long-term difficulties such as stuttering or dyslexia.

- Significant health problems that could affect the ability of the individual to benefit from intervention.

Non-organic factors

- Language used in the home, for example the amount of, nature of, mother tongue, etc., which will affect decisions about when, where or with whom (for example a bilingual co-worker) intervention takes place.
- Care-giver communication, such as the ability of the parent to interact effectively with the child or the amount of language used in a day care centre for the elderly, will again affect decisions about the focus of intervention.
- Sibling language and competition for time, which may be putting pressure on a child with slow development or with normal non-fluency and which will need to be thought about in your intervention plans.
- Social groups, school or work environments that may or may not provide additional demands on the speech and language system of your client. For example, a noisy classroom for a teacher with a voice disorder, or high demand for oral skills in a high school which a child with a stutter attends. Your decisions about possible change in your client will need to include the flexibility of these environments and their openness to change.
- Personal or emotional factors, such as awareness and sensitivity, which may work for or against the therapeutic process. For example, a hyper-anxious client with dysarthria may be unable to try out or maintain new skills in his or her normal environment, while a client who lacks aware-ness of the effect of his or her fast rate of speech on others will be unlikely to try to modify this behaviour.

**Working through the process**

*Case discussions: Adam and Charles*

*A. Nature of the language disorder*

Both children present with a developmental language delay. Byers Brown and Edwards (1989) suggest that this term, as well as 'develop-mental language disorder', is used descriptively and is not a diagnostic category itself. It includes children with some known causal factors as well as those with none. The range of language behaviours that the children show is great and difficulties may be seen in comprehension and/or expression in the realms of syntax and/or semantics and/or phonology and/or pragmatics, as well as possible problems with reading and writing.

## B. Severity

**Adam** presents with no verbal expression. He makes his needs known by pointing and producing a high pitched [e]. His parents both seem to understand and anticipate his needs and supply him with what he wants almost immediately. On the rare occasions when they are unable to guess, Adam will fling himself on the floor and have a full-blown tantrum wherever he is. His parents try to avoid this as much as possible by always carrying toys and snacks that he enjoys to try and distract him if he looks as if he may be getting frustrated. Adam's parents feel that he understands what they say within reason – he will go and get named items and show interest when they tell him where they are going – but he often appears to ignore what they ask. He plays well with cars, Lego, his bike and a football, but usually requires that his parents play with him. He is an only child.

    **Charles** also has very little verbal expression. He has a few words, recognizable to his parents, for his dog, his favourite toy (a stuffed rabbit) and his bottle, which he takes to bed. His parents describe him as easygoing and no bother. He doesn't seem to need much entertaining and will sit rocking with his rabbit for long periods. He is a fussy eater and his mother gets concerned about this. At present he will only eat bananas and Weetabix. He will suddenly go off these foods and on to another limited set. Charles's parents say that he pays very little attention to them and, while he is fairly compliant if they take him by the hand and lead him to where they want, he does not show much awareness of their language to him. He does, however, enjoy songs and sounds on television. Charles has an older brother with whom he enjoys rough and tumble play.

    You can begin to organize the information you have obtained so far. By highlighting the importance of the information through +s for significance and -s for insignificance, you can build a picture of their needs which will affect your decision making (Table 3.10).

## C. Age

Both boys are 3 years of age. However, there are differences in what might be considered the age of onset when the parents are questioned.

**Table 3.10:** Severity of symptoms for Adam and Charles

| Adam | | Charles | |
|------|------|---------|------|
| Severe symptom – | expression +++ <br> comprehension ++ | Severe symptom – | expression +++ <br> comprehension +++ |
| Parental concern +++ | | Parental concern + | |
| Child awareness ++ | | Child awareness – | |
| Affects family life ++ | | Affects family life + | |

**Adam** seemed to develop well. He was an alert baby and his motor milestones were within the early normal range: he sat alone at 5 months, was crawling at 7 months and walking at 10 months. He showed an alert interest in everything and made the expected baby cooing and babbling according to his parents. It was not till he was 2 that they began to worry about his lack of words. He had made his needs known so well without words that his parents had not really realized that he was behind until his mother took him to a mother and toddler group. She had expressed some concern to her doctor but was assured that, as everything else was coming along well, Adam would probably catch up in this area.

**Charles** had always been a good baby. He slept a lot and did not seem to demand food. He was happy to be woken and fed and would look at his mother and smile, but did not seem very interested in anything around him. His parents knew he was very different from their first child and questioned whether he was deaf. When he was 1 year old his doctor arranged for a hearing test. He responded well to visual reinforcement audiometry and he was healthy and developing well, if a little slowly, so his parents were told that there was no problem. At 2 he was saying a few words and, although he was very different from his brother, his parents accepted that he was simply slower in development and were not very concerned. When he was 3, he joined a nursery class and it was there that his lack of language became very apparent.

So, while both boys are showing a definite delay in language, it appears that this is part of a more general developmental delay for Charles. Charles's parents have been aware of a problem from an early age whereas Adam's parents have only really identified a difficulty since language should have been developing (Table 3.11).

**Table 3.11:** Age as significant for Adam and Charles

| Adam | Charles |
| --- | --- |
| Child's age + | Child's age + |
| Time between age noticed and present − | Time between age noticed and present +++ |

## D. Causal and/or maintaining factors

A few decisions can be made at present based on the information you have about the boys. But there are likely to be many more questions you will need to ask and observations you will need to make before you can feel that you know enough to be confident about causal or maintaining factors.

There seem to be few causal factors in **Adam's** case. His mother had no illnesses during pregnancy and he has had none since. His general development suggests no overt neurological problems and there is no history of speech difficulties in the family. Adam sees well and his parents feel he hears well. A simple speech discrimination test suggests that he is hearing sounds distinctively and you are not overly concerned about his hearing though you will keep an eye on this and refer him for a full hearing test if you feel it is necessary at a later date. The non-organic factors that are significant are the amount of concern expressed by his parents and the fact that Adam can obtain his needs without speech. He shows an obvious awareness and sensitivity to communication breakdown and is already manipulating his parents through his tantrums. Adam seems to be able in many areas: he plays symbolically and imaginatively, he is keen to group and match, and plays simple games of snap and pelmanism. In fact he is very capable of recalling what pictures he has recently turned over. Because of his severe expressive language difficulty, his parents don't know whether he can recall auditory information such as nursery rhymes but his mother reports that he can anticipate the actions in rhymes such as 'Ring-o-Roses'. Adam attends a nursery three afternoons a week where he seems to play well with other children.

**Charles** has a very different pattern from Adam. His mother reported a series of minor ailments during the pregnancy and an increase in blood pressure leading to inducement of the birth a week before the due date. Charles had been a good size but was slow to breathe and was in a special baby unit for a day. After that he picked up and did well. He was always a slow feeder and was often sick, but he put on weight slowly and went home from hospital a week after his birth. While he had never had any major illnesses, he often had colds and chestiness. He sat at 10 months, did not crawl but pulled himself about from 1 year. He walked at 18 months and since then has progressed well on gross motor skills. His hearing is of concern, even though he passed the early test. There is no history of speech problems in the family and his brother is doing well and has no difficulties. Non-organic factors are the lack of expectations of him in the home. Charles is somewhat repetitive in his play. He enjoys grouping and sorting objects but will do this to the exclusion of other activities. His brother says he will not play a card game with him, nor will Charles play imaginatively. He does enjoy football and running around outside, however. At nursery he is very active and enjoys the climbing frame and the bikes, but the nursery teachers find it difficult to contain him during quieter activities such as painting or stories.

There are now additional factors to add to the strengths and weaknesses of the two boys (Table 3.12), and you have reached a point where you need to use the information gathered in order to reach a decision about future management. Your options are:

- to do nothing
- to refer on
- to give a home programme
- to see for review at a later date
- to offer indirect therapy via others
- to offer direct therapy with parents only or child only
- to offer direct therapy with child and parents together

- to see for therapy occasionally
- to see for therapy regularly.

**Table 3.12:** Causative and maintenance factors for Adam and Charles

| Adam | Charles |
|---|---|
| Pregnancy factors – | Pregnancy factors + |
| Past illnesses – | Past illnesses + + |
| Neurological factors: | Neurological factors: |
|     attention – |     attention + + |
|     listening skills + |     listening skills + + + |
|     memory/learning skills – |     memory/learning skills + + |
|     development – |     development + |
|     sensory – |     sensory + + |
|     family history – |     family history – |
| Environment: | Environment: |
|     parental concern + + + |     parental concern – |
|     child awareness + + |     child awareness – |

*Collation of all the information known so far about Adam and Charles*

You now need to work through a process of considering the significance of the information you have collected. You might start by asking yourself questions and following the answers through in a logical step-by-step fashion. A flowchart such as the one developed in Figures 3.10-3.12 might be a helpful way to do this.

Question 1: Is there cause for concern in the areas investigated?

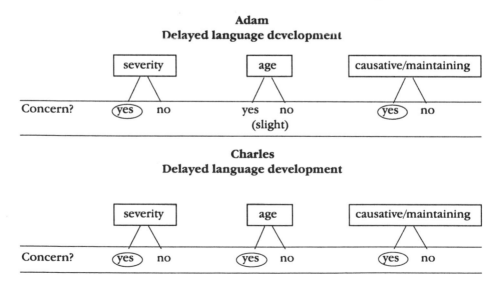

**Figure 3.10:** Is there a problem?

Question 2: In what areas are the problems located?

**Adam**
**Delayed language development**

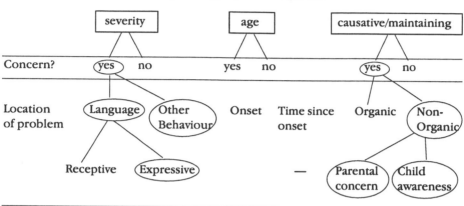

**Charles**
**Delayed language development**

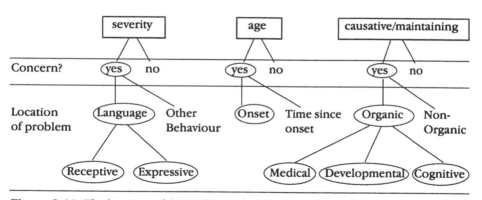

**Figure 3.11:** The location of the problems for Adam and Charles.

*General summary of the two children*

Adam's language difficulty seems to be more specifically focused on verbal expression than Charles's. Parental anxiety is the major area of concern in relation to maintaining factors, but Adam also shows a high degree of awareness and reaction to his difficulties. Although Adam is still only 3, his communicative behaviour is similar to that of a 12-18-month-old child, so it is severely delayed.

Charles's problem seems to be more pervasive and affects many more cognitive areas of behaviour than Adam's. His comprehension of language appears to be minimal and his lack of interest in communication is of concern. Charles appears to have some causative areas of significance pointing to possible neurological dysfunction.

Question 3: What is the nature of and how severe are these problems?

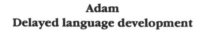

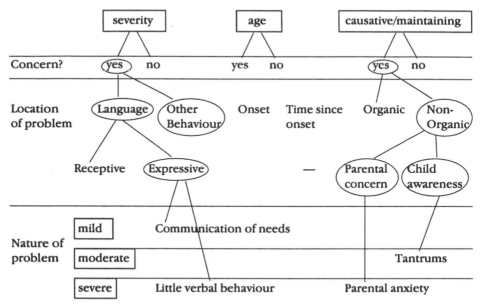

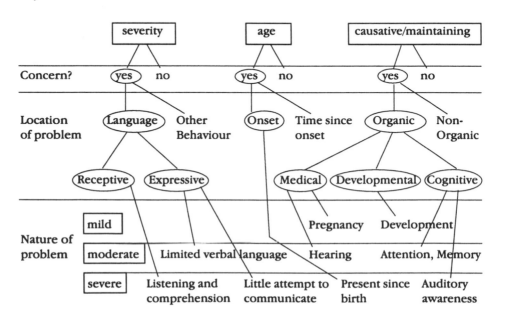

**Figure 3.12:** Nature and severity of problems for Adam and Charles.

Both children have interested and involved parents and both are of similar age.

## Decisions and prognoses

Following this careful consideration of the data, you can now make some decisions about which options to follow. You also have some ideas on the possible prognoses or long term outcomes for the two boys.
You decide that:

- Both children need some kind of intervention based on the fact that they present with severely delayed language development.
- Both need their hearing checked, but this is more immediate in Charles's case because of his lack of response to his parents' language.
- Both sets of parents are keen to be involved and specific information and ideas related to attention and listening, which is affected in both boys, will be of benefit.
- As Adam is showing frustration and developing behavioural responses to his difficulty, and as his parents show a high level of concern, you feel it is necessary to see him and his parents together on a regular basis.
- Charles has just started nursery and you decide that discussion and involvement with the staff is essential. You feel that Charles may have a more general delay and may be exhibiting some signs of a pragmatic disorder, which needs to be understood and responded to in particular ways. You decide to see him on a fortnightly basis while he is settling in and to work out with the staff a record of his communicative behaviours.
- Charles's mother is happy to keep some records of his behaviour at home to contribute to an overall understanding of his problems.
- You feel that Adam has a good chance of showing rapid change with the involvement of his parents and because he has a more specific problem. Charles is likely to show a gradual improvement in all areas, including language, as part of a general development of neurological maturity.

This same careful analysis of information can be applied to any person with any disorder and leads to decisions that are based on knowledge and facts. Other factors, of course, may be part of the equation, such as the policy of your employer, the nature of your timetable, the ability of other professionals to be involved, and so on.

As you become involved with the client (in this case the child and his family) you need to adjust flexibly to what you are learning through the ongoing process of assessment and reassessment, negotiation with those involved and the outcomes your intervention is aimed towards.

Having discussed the process of assessment and decision making in detail, in the next chapter we go on to consider the process of therapy. This will move on from the base of the hypotheses and decisions made but will keep returning to these and to the whole assessment process as a means of checking its effectiveness and direction. The purpose of assessment is discovery while the purpose of therapy is to bring about change. Change will lead to new discoveries, so while therapy is being undertaken, assessment and the gaining of information and knowledge will be continuing hand-in-hand.

# Chapter 4
# Therapy: Process and Practice

You sit on the floor with a child and from a big bag you pull interesting objects which you then cause to disappear under a cloth, only to make them re-emerge and jump into the child's hand. As you do this you make the noise of the object – a chuffing train, a whistling bird, a buzzing bee. The child delightedly hides the objects behind his back and you pretend to look for them. You 'call' each item by making its noise. You then find the items behind the child, who laughs and gives them up as you hold out your hand and make the noise for each. Is this therapy?

You sit at a table in your clinic with a child and her mother. You put on the table a series of pictures and encourage the child to find the sequence that tells the story. You then ask the child to tell her mother the story. As the three of you work together on this, you comment on the pictures that the child seems to find difficult, 'Oh, this is where they are packing to go on holiday. I can see dad putting the case in the car'. You remind the child of aspects of the pictures that she has missed, not in a judgemental way but in a way designed to engage her interest in providing information, 'Did you tell your mother about the dog jumping into the car?' (said quietly so the information is not yet shared by the child's mother). Is this therapy?

You sit quietly in a room next to an elderly lady. She is trying to tell you about her son who has moved to another town. She makes many false starts, she chooses and rejects the words or sounds that make up the words she is trying to utter. She gestures and points. You feed back what you have heard; you ask for more information about the place; you follow her pointing hand and suggest an area of the country it might be in; you offer a phoneme as a cue for a town in that locality. Eventually, she is able to produce a word close enough to the name of a town that you know where he is living. You comment on her persistence and her ability to get the information across and she looks relieved and more relaxed. Is this therapy?

## Defining therapy

What has been described above can be loosely termed methods. Methods are what you do but they do not by themselves constitute therapy. So what is therapy? Byng and Black (1995: 305) suggest that in language remediation therapy is 'a combination of the task, the materials and the psycholinguistic concepts conveyed through the task, and the therapist/patient interaction'. To try and understand what therapy is composed of, you may find the iceberg model shown in Figure 4.1 helpful.

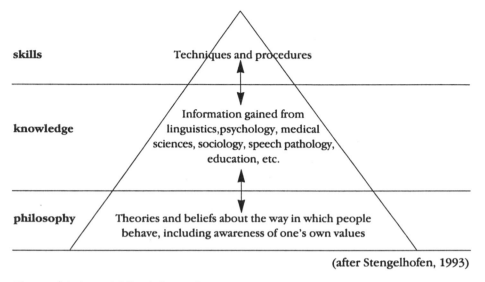

(after Stengelhofen, 1993)

**Figure 4.1:** A model for defining therapy.

The pinnacle of this iceberg, the *skills* level, is the techniques and procedures such as have been described on the previous page. These are on the surface and are those aspects of the process seen by others. Comments from those who do not understand the profession, such as 'Oh, anyone can talk to an old lady' or 'Why do you need a degree to teach you to play with children?', stem from an ignorance of what is under the surface of the water, of what underpins procedures which look so easy.

The next level under that of skills, and from which skills evolve, is that of *knowledge*. It is impossible to decide what you should do with a person in therapy without a sound knowledge of the linguistic and other difficulties that are present, the approaches recommended in the literature for understanding and treating these disorders, and the developmental and psychological factors inherent in the person who is in therapy. You develop your competence in this area from the linguistics, medical sciences, psychology, sociology, education and speech pathology that you learn as part of your university training.

The deepest level of the iceberg is that of *philosophy*. Your decisions about how you will use your knowledge and develop techniques of therapy are driven by your thinking about how people learn, what motivates them, how they come to see the world as they do, why they behave in certain ways. Equally important are your own beliefs and values and how they influence your actions and decisions.

Based on this model, therapy can be defined as behaviours that come about through a combination of philosophy, knowledge and skills, all three of which influence and are influenced by the others through processes of monitoring and of reflection.

## The levels of the therapy process

We shall now look more closely at each of the three levels of the therapy process, starting with the deepest and least obvious level, that of philosophy. This is the level that can so often be unrecognized and neglected, yet it may drive decisions and procedures. It must therefore be made explicit so that it can be utilized purposefully in therapeutic decision making.

### Philosopy

1. Observation and imitation, modelling of behaviour, feedback, reinforcement, reward and punishment are all based on the idea that behaviour can be learned when it has certain consequences, and a therapist can aid or manipulate this learning by carefully monitoring and contingently reacting to a client's behaviour. The principles of *learning theory*, and particularly of *behaviourism,* have had an enormous influence on the profession and the therapy that is offered. Your decisions about whether or not to adopt a teaching role, how structured or unstructured your therapy programme will be and how to manage issues of general behaviour will most likely stem from your awareness and utilization of learning theory.

2. Attitudes and beliefs, values and prejudice, and the influence of these on learning and thinking and on the way people behave form the basis of *cognitive theories* which underlie many of the techniques you might use to help your clients develop realistic self-awareness.

3. A belief in the capability of your client to change and develop, to make decisions and to come to his or her own solutions, as well as approaches that enhance your client's self-esteem and realistic self-concept, will be based on your own understanding of theories of personality, particularly those of the *humanistic school*. Decisions about how much to involve your client as a partner in the therapeutic process and how directive or non-directive your approaches will be may stem from this underlying philosophy.

4. An awareness of the influence of society and of various groups and interpersonal relationships on an individual's behaviour, and an understanding of contexts and their influence on behaviour, form the basis of *social theories* which drive decisions about where and with whom therapy will take place.

5. Whether you believe people are genetically programmed to behave in certain ways (such as to develop language) or whether you think they learn to become the people they are through interaction with the

environment, will influence and bias your thinking about an individual's behaviour and the intervention you might offer. This is known as the *nature-nurture* debate, which is still discussed in the speech and language area in relation to how much of language acquisition is innate and how much is encouraged through child-care-giver interaction (see books such as that by Pinker (1994) and Marschark et al. (1997) for further discussion of this area).

There are probably many more underlying philosophies which direct and influence the behaviour of the therapist and his or her understanding of the people with whom therapy will be conducted. Those outlined above have all had a clear influence over the years on the way speech and language therapy is conducted. Certain philosophies hold sway at certain times – they grow out of the knowledge, beliefs and expectations of the society in which you live. You must remember that much of your perception of human behaviour is based on Western European ideals and must be critically examined when it conflicts with the philosophies of clients who may come from other cultural and social backgrounds. Philosophical concepts and ideas are open to modification and change as new knowledge and new beliefs emerge.

**Knowledge**

In Chapters 1 and 3, the areas of knowledge that are used as the basis of exploration and understanding of the speech and language difficulties which affect clients were discussed. So in this chapter we will consider how a knowledge of treatment approaches may be used to guide your decisions on what to do. For example:

1. In the field of stuttering, there are two main schools of approach, which have been termed 'stutter more fluently' and 'speak more fluently' (Gregory, 1979). The techniques used within these schools vary quite considerably, though many therapists nowadays use ideas and approaches stemming from both. A knowledge of what each school has to offer and how this might relate to the nature of the client's symptoms is essential for considered decision making by the therapist.
   - The 'stutter more fluently' approach suggests that chronic stuttering can only be modified within the framework of changing the whole person. The person who stutters must learn to accept his role of stutterer and can work to modify his or her speech, but can rarely eliminate the stuttering. Van Riper (1973) was a major proponent of this approach and his ideas are still used extensively in stuttering therapy.
   - The 'speak more fluently' approach teaches the person to control output by modifying speech to such an extent that the stuttering is not observable by the listener. Ingham (1984) argues in favour of the techniques associated with this approach.

2. Howard and Hatfield (1987) suggest that there are a number of different schools of aphasia therapy. Decisions about which approach is likely to be most beneficial for the person you are working with will need to be based on a clear understanding of what each entails. Some of these schools are mentioned below to give you an idea of how they might influence the type of therapy you offer:

   - The didactic school views remediation as a process of teaching (or reteaching) skills that have been lost based on a developmental framework.
   - The stimulation school targets those language behaviours which remain intact but inaccessible in aphasia by appropriate and often intensive stimulation – particularly of the auditory system.
   - The pragmatic school believes that the needs of the client with aphasia are for improved communication through the encouragement of the use of unimpaired abilities such as gesture, drawing, etc.
   - The cognitive neuropsychological school attempts to understand the difficulties seen in people with aphasia by reference to information processing models. Treatment focuses on encouraging the client to use those psycholinguistic skills that are intact to compensate for areas of difficulty with a view to improving communicative competence.

3. In child language therapy there are numerous approaches which can be considered by the therapist:

   - The whole language approach (Alcorn et al., 1995) assumes that learning of language is through exposure to an environment where the child is stimulated with appropriately chosen and directed language games and activities. The need of the child to communicate drives the choice of activities, and parents and therapists provide models of the way in which the child might use language to achieve his or her ends.
   - An articulatory approach based on learning theory principles may be used when children have a known or suspected articulatory difficulty and need to be exposed to the skill of production. It is assumed that motor movements can improve with practice and that articulatory competence can be affected through drills. This is a tried and tested approach suitable for some clients and can be found in books such as that by Van Riper and Emerick (1984).
   - Non-directive, child-centred therapy is based on the person-centred philosophy of Carl Rogers (1951) and is based on the belief that children will learn if they are allowed the freedom in a safe environment to explore and develop at their own pace.
   - Associated with the non-directive approach and fitting comfortably into this philosophy is Vygotsky's concept of the 'Zone of Proximal Development' (Geekie and Raban, 1994: 159), where the child is

offered models of behaviour which will challenge but not overface his or her desire to learn.

- The metaphonological approach (Howell and Dean, 1994) for children with phonological disorders uses a cognitive and linguistic framework to help children to understand and change their manner of production. Helping children to make meaningful contrasts in their speech to convey appropriate messages is the hoped for outcome.
- The psycholinguistic approach (Stackhouse and Wells, 1997) uses an information-processing model to encourage the therapist to hypothesize about the nature of the child's difficulty and to systematically assess and come to understand each level of linguistic behaviour. Armed with this knowledge, the therapist should be able to target the most appropriate linguistic level for remediation.

These, and other, approaches are available for you as therapist to use, and the more you know and understand the various philosophies underlying them and the skills and procedures of which they are composed, the wider will be your choice. Your decision about which approach to choose should be based on what you and your client have agreed seems to be best at this time. It may be that your basic underlying philosophy will sway you towards a particular approach. You must ask yourself 'Is this the right one for this person at this time?' Only your knowledge of yourself, your client and the options available can prevent you from making the wrong choice of therapy. But sometimes you just will not know whether this client will respond to a certain kind of approach. In such cases, careful explanation of why you are trying a certain approach and what criteria you will use to decide whether to proceed or to change it is necessary. Remember that a hypothesis-driven approach is necessary in therapy – 'If we try X then Y should happen'. If it does not happen, then a new hypothesis is in order. Many therapy practices that work well arise out of cautious trial-and-error approaches.

## Skills

When you see someone who is very skilled working, you will often exclaim at how easy it all looks. The session flows smoothly, the client is engaged and interested, the tasks are meaningful in relation to the client's age, sex, culture, disability, etc. What skills are being used? Stengelhofen (1993: 150) suggests that the skills shown in Figure 4.2 are important in clinical management.

### Decision-making skills

In the previous chapter, we discussed decision-making skills in relation to whether or not to offer therapy. In this chapter, we are interested in how a task is chosen. Remember that the choice of task must be based on the aims and objectives for this client. Once you have decided these (which we shall be looking at later in this chapter), the skill of planning the task is embarked upon:

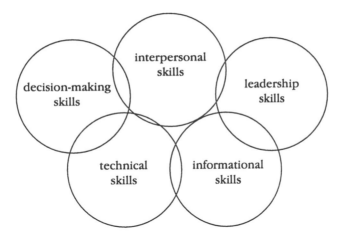

(after Stengelhofen, 1993)

The skills are represented as overlapping circles to suggest that, while they may be defined separately, they depend on and support each other.

**Figure 4.2:** Skills in clinical management.

- You might see a therapist engaged in tasks with a child and parent, such as blowing bubbles through a straw, playing with a toy garage and cars, arranging pictures into a sequence and retelling the story.
- You may see him or her having a conversation, asking the client to think of as many items within one semantic category as possible within a time limit or drawing pictures of items to be bought in a shop.
- The therapist might be engaging a group in a game of 'wink murder', asking members to solve a problem together or planning and going ahead with an outing of some kind.

How is the therapist making decisions about what activities to do in therapy? How has he or she decided whether to see this client individually or in a group or with the family? To make these decisions you might need to be competent at, for example:

- negotiating with the client/s
- considering all the options available
- excluding ideas that are inappropriate
- taking into account the nature of the materials related to the disabilities of the client/s
- considering the influence of environmental factors.

*Interpersonal skills*

Developing a good rapport, being sensitive to the client's needs, knowing when fatigue or emotion are taking over and how to deal with them when they do, knowing how to alter the pace, tone or level of the activity are all part of being competent in the area of interpersonal skills. Dryden (1990) asked authorities in counselling what qualities an effective therapist needs within the therapy regime offered by a particular approach. Many of these authors agreed that the qualities were:

- the core counselling qualities of genuineness, warmth and empathy, which are based on the skills of observing, listening and responding appropriately
- sensitivity to others
- respect for clients
- a credulous approach (that is, accept what the client offers as truth for him or her)
- self-awareness
- a desire to go on developing and broadening life experiences
- trustworthiness and dependability.

Therapeutic relationships are built and sustained through informed involvement of the therapist. They do not just 'happen'. You have to work hard to reach a competent level in the ability to build rapport with clients.

Another set of interpersonal skills which are constantly in use by the speech and language clinician are those loosely termed 'social skills'. These are based on a sensitivity to what is appropriate in a given situation and knowing how to modify your own behaviour when in this situation. So you might:

- adopt a quiet listening role when negotiating how a teacher might help a child in his or her classroom, adapting your posture, facial expressions and proximity to convey the acceptance of the teacher's dominant role in classroom management
- be assertive and confident when providing models of therapy techniques to clients and their carers in the clinic using clear speech, adequate volume and well-controlled gestures and movements
- be calm and slow moving when presented with a highly anxious individual, reducing eye contact and keeping a fair distance from the client so as not to be seen as a threat
- show enthusiasm and excitement when playing a game with a child, getting on the same physical level as the child and using a lot of eye contact, facial expression and increased intonation
- adopt the rules of reduced eye contact or increased formality that are expected when with a client from a different cultural background.

As you can see, the ability to modify behaviours such as facial expression, proximity, etc., in appropriate ways is directly related to the development of the core qualities as specified by Dryden above.

*Leadership skills*

These skills will be discussed in Chapter 5 in relation to working with groups. It is important, however, to consider them in this chapter as well, as the management of group therapy, family therapy, working with groups of carers and so on depend on good leadership skills. To be good in a group setting, you must:

- maintain all the attitudes mentioned above in relation to interpersonal skills
- understand the way in which groups influence behaviour
- know about leadership styles and be clear about your role
- know about roles that people in groups might play and how to monitor individuals' inputs into the group.

Fawcus (1992) reminds us that, whether we take account of the psychosocial factors in a group or not, the mere fact of being part of a group will have a positive or negative effect on the attitudes and feelings of the participants. It is very important therefore that you know and understand what the dynamics of groups are and what role you will play as leader.

*Technical skills*

What are the technical skills of a speech and language clinician? In our profession they are less easy to identify and isolate than in some other professions where particular accurate measures might be relatively straightforward, for example measuring the length of one leg against another, or the height to weight ratio of a person, etc. Below we have identified a few of the technical skills in speech and language therapy, but you could probably add many, many more.

- Measurement in speech and language therapy requires a knowledge of the standardized, or preferred, way of administering a procedure and the standard way of recording the information. So reading and understanding manuals associated with testing procedures would be a way of acquiring this skill.
- Manipulating the switches on a tape reorder or a video recorder and understanding how to get the best audio or video recording (taking into account light, ambient noise, etc.) is an important skill.
- Transcribing linguistic information in a standard form – using conventions for orthographic or phonetic transcription – is a very skilled job based on much practice.
- Managing the testing or teaching equipment in the therapy space so that it is accessible but not distracting helps the ease and flow of the therapy session.

- Choosing, making or adapting materials to suit the client/s and their level of ability is a skill based on a strong knowledge base.
- Modelling wanted behaviours, cueing and reinforcing to channel or modify clients' attempts to reach a planned goal are skills based on knowledge of goalsetting and behaviour modification.
- Using counselling skills such as attending behaviours, paraphrasing, reflecting, summarizing, etc., to encourage clients to feel able to discuss information openly.
- Recording of behaviour and activities as they occur in the therapy sessions, using appropriate and relatively quick scoring methods to keep records of outcomes of your interventions, is a vital skill, again based on knowledge of anticipated goals.

### Informational skills

When you meet a client or his family, the teacher of a child with speech and language difficulties or a voluntary group wanting to know and understand the nature of language problems, you need to call on the skills of offering appropriate information. When you write a report or give verbal feedback on a client to another professional, or you become involved with setting up a programme for a child at school linked in with the national curriculum, you need a different set of informational skills. When you offer suggestions for tasks to be attempted at home or in other non-clinical settings, you are using another set of these skills. So you need to develop:

- a good basis of knowledge in the particular area
- a good understanding of what level of information is appropriate
- an ability to choose words carefully in order to present the information in a clear and concise way, i.e. good spoken language skills
- good written language skills in order to present reports, etc. clearly
- an ability to provide information in ways other than spoken or written English if your client/s cannot comprehend this – so use of mime, sign, modelling, pictures, symbols may be needed
- an awareness of the effects of your information-offering style on the client/s.

Heron (1990:32) suggests there is a directive continuum along which any prescriptive intervention (which is what information giving is) can be placed. This has five grades from mild to strong which are

(a) suggest
(b) propose
(c) advise
(d) persuade
(e) command.

Your own awareness of the 'tone' in which you offer information is essential if you wish clients and others to listen to, remember and respond to what you have to offer.

## The therapy plan

Armed with your philosophy, knowledge and skills, you are now ready to start the process of converting theory into practice via the therapy plan. Every good worker requires a plan in order to complete a task. If you think of an area of work such as the clothing industry, you can see that it would be in chaos if there was no idea of how the clothes would look or the steps needed to achieve a pre-designed garment. In speech and language therapy, simply doing tasks, playing games or being nice to people is not enough. You need to have a way of focusing your thinking and channelling it into a working document – a blueprint for the activities you will undertake. To do this, you might work systematically through a flowchart such as the one in Figure 4.3. The words used in this flowchart may differ for different people, for example the word 'goal' may be used instead of 'objective' and so on, but the principles will be universal.

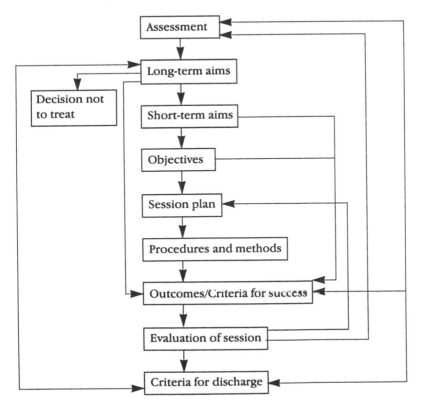

**Figure 4.3:** A flowchart of the therapy-planning process.

*Assessment* has had a chapter of its own because it is so important. It is the starting point for your plan. But it is also a point to which you constantly return. Therapy can only proceed successfully if you are regularly using what you are learning about the client to review and reconsider the original decisions you made about his or her difficulties.

*Long-term aims* are based on what you know from the assessment and what this tells you about where the client might be at the point of discharge. This requires an understanding of the nature of the condition and its likely course and factors that lie within the domain of the client (e.g. age, personality and support from others, which were discussed at length in the section on decision making). It also requires knowledge of the constraints of working practice and practical details, such as availability of transport, distance of the clinic from the client's home, space, time available, and so on. For some clients you will be aiming to develop language skills to a level where they are age appropriate, while with others you will hope for communicative competence within the constraints mentioned above. For some you might be looking to maintain skills for as long as possible and offering alternatives when necessary; for yet others you will be providing carers with as much information and support as possible to deal with the long-term language problems presented by their spouse, relative or friend.

These long-term *intentions* would be written as a list of hoped-for outcomes covering all aspects of the management of this individual such as:

- what you hope will be the linguistic changes
- what you hope will be the changes in other related behaviours (learning ability, play, etc.)
- what you hope will be the attitude changes
- what you hope will be changes in the social or family systems
- what you hope will be the changes in the personal and emotional well-being of the individual.

*Short-term aims* will relate directly to the long-term aims but will 'chunk' the timescale of treatment into manageable pieces and will identify where the therapist and client will hope to be within a certain short timescale, such as six weeks, four weeks or a school term or semester. You will need to decide what are the priorities for work at this particular time based on the long-term hoped for outcomes. These will be negotiated with your client, his or her family, the teaching staff, the ward staff or involved others – you cannot make these decisions on your own. So you will take one or two of the above list and reduce the overall aim into a sequence of subaims.

Each set of short-term aims should hopefully be a step up the ladder to the long-term outcomes. The end of the period assigned to reach the short-term aims will be a time for reflecting on progress so far and recycling back to additional assessment or exploration of the problem if necessary.

*Objectives* are the more tangible outcomes – the actual behaviours or feelings or attitudes – that can be measured to help you and your client identify change. They are the carefully analysed sequence of steps that will guide the client to the outcome.

## Case discussion: Peter

Peter is a 40-year-old man who was head-injured in a fall. He has particular difficulty in maintaining a steady rate of speech. With excessive speed comes elision of syllables and, at times, whole words, which makes Peter very difficult to understand. He is having difficulty monitoring this behaviour. Your short-term aim in relation to this linguistic problem is to improve Peter's ability to recognize fast and unintelligible speech.

**Aim:** To improve Peter's monitoring skills by helping him recognize when his speech has become very fast.

*Objectives:* That Peter will:

- learn to use a word-per-minute count to measure rate of speech
- discriminate fast and slow speech of a variety of speakers via tape recordings with 100 per cent accuracy
- identify which of his own spoken sentences are fast, using tape recordings of his speech
- measure his own rate of speech.

At the end of the period of therapy, you should be able to agree with Peter that these objectives have or have not been met and decide what to focus on next.

### Session plan

Some examples of session plans will be given at the end of this chapter. The session plan starts with the aims and objectives for the particular day. These will be based on the short-term aims and will be even more precise and detailed than those suggested above. The session plan contains a list of the actual procedures you will undertake that move the process from the idea to the action. It will also contain suggestions for methods and materials needed to accomplish the procedures.

*Procedures* are the course of action that will turn the concepts of goals or objectives into tangible activities. Procedures are not arbitrary, they are in fact tightly tied to the aims and objectives and as such are not simply intuitive or random. However, the procedures are that aspect of the therapy process that can be called 'creative'. When a therapist is working well with a client or group of clients, using his or her knowledge and skills effectively, and is sure and clear about the underlying philosophy that is driving the process, we are likely to say that what we are seeing is a very *creative* person.

But what is creativity? Edward de Bono (1985), in interviews with creative people from many walks of life, found that there are numerous different ways of allowing creative ideas to evolve. Among them are the following:

- Put everything you know into 'the pot' (your mind, a piece of paper, a discussion with a colleague), and through this process of brain-storming ideas will evolve.
- Allow yourself to be completely preoccupied with the ideas in order to arrive at solutions.
- Put the knowledge and information you have into groups and categories and take note of any gaps.
- Think freely and widely – what do you still need to know? What approaches would be possible given this client's age, interests, linguistic level, home situation? What are your own biases in therapy and are you being influenced by these? What ideas and suggestions have been given to you by others? What therapy ideas have you read about that might be useful here?

This process of thinking loosely and allowing all thought to be accepted and considered is the best way to come to that point of 'Eureka', where you suddenly get an idea or see much more clearly where you are going.

### Case discussion: George

Imagine you are faced with the need to develop some tasks in order to meet the objective that your client George, a 60-year-old who has aphasia, will begin to initiate more conversation.

*Experiences* First, you may think about your own experiences in initiating conversations. What makes it easy or difficult to start? What do you do when you enter a conversation? How do other people that you know initiate conversations? Have you seen other people of this age or other people with aphasia in conversation? How do they cope?

*Knowledge* Next you might look at the linguistic literature on conversational exchange to see what is known about the processing needed to initiate language and the skills used to start conversations. You may wish to read the neuropsychological literature to find out what is known about the effects of brain injury on initiation of behaviour. You now turn to your knowledge of this particular man. What is the extent and location of his brain injury? How severe is his linguistic loss? What was he like before the stroke? Did he enjoy and engage in conversation? Who does he have now to talk to? Does this person enjoy and want to be engaged in conversation? What are the hurdles he will need to overcome if he is to participate in conversation with another?

*Perception* The way you look at and make sense of this information is biased by your own experiences and values. You perceive the problem in a particular way. The more you can be aware of and avoid thinking in a channelled fashion, the more creative will be your ideas. You might wish to share ideas for therapy for this man with a friend. Ask questions of your friend as if she were the client. 'How would you feel if I asked you to tell me about your family? What would you do in a situation where you had to engage a stranger in conversation?'

Remember that there are no rights or wrongs in this sort of decision making. There are a number of alternative procedures that you and your client are free to try out. Once you have embarked on the tasks you are still not bound to carry them through to the bitter end. Think of yourself and your client as scientists formulating and testing out new hypotheses about what works and what doesn't, about what might be useful in generating change (Kelly, 1963).

## Methods and materials

Each step of your overall session plan takes the process to a more microscopic level. Methods may be seen therefore as an orderly set of actions based on the overall procedure.

### Case Discussion: George, continued

*Objectives for a session with George*

By the end of this session George will have:

- gained my attention by any means possible at least four times
- produced some 'opening' utterance or gesture on each occasion.

*Procedures*

1. Explain the nature of the task to George.
2. Look at the articles on gardening that he said he would bring.
3. Wait – do not ask questions. This is to give George time to initiate.
4. Respond immediately to any attention getting device – George might point, move the paper, produce a non-verbal sound (throat clearing).

5. Respond appropriately to any initiations made by George and paraphrase any verbal attempts.
6. Record George's behaviour and discuss this with him.

*Methods*

The numbering applies to the procedure to which these methods are attached:

1. Explanation must:
   • focus on idea of starting off
   • reinforce idea that he is more knowledgeable than I am in this area
   • reinforce that he can indicate need for help if necessary.
2. Read paragraph from articles aloud to focus George's attention.
3. Use non-verbal reinforcements to encourage him to find something he wishes to draw my attention to (nod, smile, indicate page).
4. If he seems unable to start a conversation, consider:
   • guiding his hand to a point on the page
   • underlining the main points on the page
   • giving alternatives – 'this or this'
   • asking direct questions if he is not forthcoming
   • if he finds it easy, move on to general gardening topics, i.e. remove the visual prompt provided by the articles.
5. Reinforce by continuing on topic he has introduced or by paraphrasing what he has said, or by giving a general comment on the area he has indicated.
6. Measure outcomes by rating 1 to 4:
   • 1 for spontaneous initiations
   • 2 for non-verbal prompts
   • 3 for verbal prompts
   • 4 for need to ask questions.

As you can see the methods are far more detailed than the procedures. It is recommended that you use this level of detail if you are insecure about what you are doing. As you become more confident, you can reduce the detail and write procedures and not methods. Experienced clinicians will be able to carry a set of aims and objectives in their heads and the procedures will come automatically as the session unfolds.

One of the outcomes of carefully thinking about methods is the development of *flexibility*. This means the ability to adapt and respond, relative to the immediate needs of the client. As you can see from the examples above, method 4 gives a range of prompts to use if George is having difficulties and an idea for moving to more spontaneous conversation should he find the task easy. To be flexible you need therefore to have a good understanding of the steps you will take to reach the goal and the prompts and cues which are appropriate and necessary to get there. You must also have a good idea of what is next in line in the overall programme (the short-term and long-term aims and objectives) so you can move up a level if necessary. Every clinician will have experienced times when a client has shown such variability that an impossible task one week is completed with ease the following week. Building flexibility into the methods is the way for an inexperienced clinician to deal with this.

## Materials

Materials would appear to be straightforward, but of course they are not. George has said he would bring some gardening articles with him. But what if he forgets? And what will you do about his poor eyesight? Where will you position the magazine to accommodate his inclination to neglect one side? A young child in therapy will need materials that will gain his or her interest, that will make the appropriate sounds, that are not in any way ambiguous. You will have to arrange to have other distractions out of sight, to reduce noise levels, etc. Will you need a video for work with a mother? Will you ask her to play with her son, and what will you suggest they play with? Will she be bringing anything from home or will you use what you have?

You can see that careful planning, time to gather what you need and creative and flexible thinking are essential elements of the therapy process.

## Outcomes/criteria for success

The question to ask of yourself and your client is 'Have the objectives been met?' However, other questions will follows this: 'How much help or cueing was needed?', 'What length of time was there before a response occurred?', 'What precision accompanied the activity?' So, if you are to have a clear idea of the usefulness of the therapy session, you need to specify at the outset what level of achievement is to be expected. If the main focus at this time in therapy is a change in attitude or feeling on the part of the client, it is less easy to be specific but still possible to consider some rating or measure of attitude change.

You can use a framework such as the one in Figure 4.4 to help you decide how to specify outcomes.

A recent discussion section in the Royal College of Speech and Language Therapists' Bulletin took up the issue of outcome measures and warned against trying to be too global, that is, covering everything possible in one measure. Global measures of change in clients, such as the Functional Independence Measure (FIM), which attempt to provide criteria for behaviour in a wide variety of domains, are proving to be

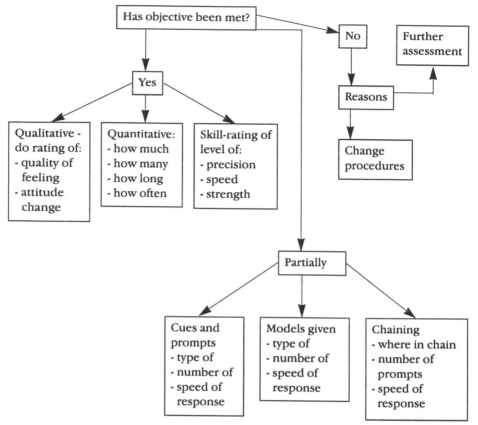

**Figure 4.4:** A flowchart to guide consideration of outcomes of therapy.

problematic in the areas of validity and of identifying change over time (Rossiter, 1997). However, it is important to consider change, not only in the domain of language, which may well be our chief concern as clinicians, but also in such areas as client wellbeing or distress (Enderby and John, 1997). Enderby and John suggest therapy outcome measures (TOM), which they have developed and which give a six-point rating scale in each of the domains of impairment, disability, handicap and wellbeing/distress. But you must also consider a number of different ways of measuring (above and beyond a rating scale) which may be through a range of different methods such as:

- retesting of previously tested areas
- further recordings and transcriptions of these to identify change
- use of a number of charts and rating scales – either published ones or those devised for this client
- client satisfaction measures
- satisfaction of involved others
- reported change by others in language, or school behaviour, etc.

*Evaluation of session*

Your evaluation should not only take into account the meeting of criteria as specified above, it should also cover less measurable aspects such as:
- did it meet the client's expectations?
- was the client interested and engaged?
- were involved others welcomed and included?
- was the setting comfortable?
- were the materials appropriate?
- was the pacing about right?
- was the overall timing about right?
- were you confident/at ease/comfortable?
- did you meet your own expectations?
- what could have been improved?
- what went better than expected?
- what have you learned that will guide ideas for the next session?

*Criteria for discharge*

These will arise from the assessment and the setting of long-term aims. However, they too are fluid and can change as you and the client get further into therapy. So it is important to bear these in mind when you evaluate how the therapy is going. Your client too may change in his or her expectations over time and may not feel the need to continue to the criteria originally set. So apart from obvious reasons for discharge, such as a client moving away, you can list:

- satisfactory achievement of long-term aims
- mutually agreed discharge before aims met
- other agencies taking over the client management, e.g. the special needs team in a school or the community team for adults with learning difficulties, etc.
- referral to another professional or to another speech and language clinician for a different therapy approach.

# The therapist in therapy

We have talked about therapy as being an agent of change in the client. But it also changes the therapist. You cannot engage in a therapeutic relationship with a client without this influencing you. You will experience a range of emotions as your client gets involved in tasks or discussions and as he or she experiences emotions such as pleasure or fear or anger. Certain clients will cause you to feel uncomfortable or anxious, with others you will be relaxed and comfortable. Some may be very like you in terms of interests and background, some may be very different. You may be reminded of people you know by an action or mannerism, a tone of voice or a turn of phrase. These reminders may be painful or pleasant, they may help you to feel confident and able, or you may be suddenly overcome by feelings of inferiority or insignificance.

It is important for you to realize that you are not alone. Everyone working closely with other people will experience a range of feelings. You need to acknowledge and accept them, to make them explicit to yourself and try to understand them.

> To try and understand oneself is not simply an interesting pastime, it is a necessity of life. In order to plan ... and to make choices, we have to be able to anticipate our behaviour in future situations. This makes self-knowledge a practical guide, not a self-indulgence. (Bannister, 1982: 202)

Self-examination can be threatening and it is often helpful to turn to another. In many speech and language therapy settings, supervision is provided to enable therapists to engage in discussion about clients, about the therapy they are offering, about their own feelings of ability or inadequacy, and so on, in a safe environment with a colleague. If this isn't an option, there are numerous books you can turn to to help you consider:

- what sort of a person you are – your underlying philosophy of life
- what are your strengths and weaknesses
- what needs are you fulfilling in therapy. Maslow (1968 in Leahy, 1995) suggests that there is a hierarchy of needs for all human beings of which the need for love and belongingness, that for esteem and that of self-fulfilment would be potentially met for the therapist in a therapy relationship
- what beliefs and attitudes bias or guide your therapy
- what personal relationships are potentially likely to intrude into the therapy situation
- what from your past life may be influencing the way you feel about this client.

And more – the list could go on. And why is it done? Roberta Green, a speech and language clinician, puts forward reasons why regular reflection about work is important (Green, 1992: 22):

- to help therapists deal with issues relating to their involvement with clients and with the personal and professional difficulties which can arise from this
- to protect the interests of clients and ensure that therapists are supported to do this
- to offer support to therapists and detect early signs of difficulties
- to challenge therapists on their work practices in a supportive, trusting environment.

We have now considered what therapy is, the framework on which you might construct your therapy, the way in which you go about planning your sessions and the processes that you go through as you develop your role as a speech and language clinician. Your primary aim must be to provide a facilitative context in which your clients can change in a positive direction.

## Using the process – therapy plans

Three clients have been selected as examples of the process of planning and decision making. They have been chosen to represent three different age groups and three different disorders. You are of course aware that each client is individual, and what you plan to do for one is never the same as what you plan for another. However, each plan builds on knowledge gained in preparation of other plans and work with one client feeds into work with another. However different clients may be, there are aspects of their assessment and therapy that can be transferred from one case to another. Hopefully, looking at plans conceived for the following three individuals will therefore give food for thought for any other clients you may see. The philosophy and knowledge on which work with these clients may be based, the aims and objectives for assessment and therapy, some possible therapy tasks and some realistic outcomes will be documented, in the hope that this will make explicit some of the information provided in this and other chapters of the book.

### Case discussion: Client 1 – Imran

Imran first came to the attention of the speech and language therapist when he entered a school for physically handicapped children at the age of four and a half years. He had spent his early years in his home country of Pakistan and his family had settled in this country six months previously. Imran's father spoke good English, he had a number of relatives settled in the UK and he had visited them regularly while preparing the ground for his own emigration. He shared the ownership of a convenience store with a cousin and worked long hours building up the business. Imran's mother spoke very little English. She lived in the home of one of the cousins, so had a great deal of support with Imran's care. Because of the close family network, she had had little contact with people outside the home until Imran started school. She also had two other younger children to care for. Neither of these children had any obvious developmental problems.

### Client 2 – David

David was seen in a community clinic by the speech and language therapist when he was 13 years of age. He had been referred by a specialist speech and language therapist in dysfluency following a week-long intensive stuttering group in the summer. David had been referred to the group by his school, as they had recognized a difficulty with his fluency. During the intensive week, it was felt that David's dysfluency was part of a more general language difficulty that had not been picked up by the school. David was seen by his teachers as being a slow learner with reading, writing and maths problems, but language problems had not been identified until the fluency difficulty had been noticed.

## Client 3 – Mary

Mary is a 35-year-old teacher who had been referred to speech and language therapy by the ear, nose and throat consultant for voice therapy. She had received a series of eight therapy sessions and her voice had become much stronger. She was aware of what she needed to do to prevent vocal abuse at school and how to look after her voice generally. Following a period of three months without therapy she had returned to a review appointment and had requested some additional help. She had again been losing her voice at the end of the day, even though she felt she had been careful not to misuse it. It was agreed that she would have a further four sessions.

### Philosophy of treatment

Each of these clients presents with a set of problems that need to be dealt with differently and from a different philosophical base.

Imran needs to be helped to develop skills necessary for communication, so an approach that will enhance his development and encourage his involvement was taken. The therapist realises that a combination of underlying theories will be needed. One of these will be a learning theory approach that will focus the therapist on seeking out what may be reinforcing to Imran and what may need to be controlled in the environment to stimulate him to learn. The other will be a child-centred approach, which will cause the therapist to be alert to Imran's needs, his fears and his desire to explore. Also the therapist is aware of the effect that entry into school and the removal of Imran from the family may have on the family system. She needs to be conversant with a systems approach to understand the relationships between all family members, Imran and his difficulties, the school and the possible effects of therapy on the family.

David, as an adolescent who is capable of working alongside the therapist, needs a different approach. He may possibly respond to a cognitive-behavioural philosophy, which will engage him in a joint venture with the therapist. This underlying theory will encourage the therapist to help David explore how his attitudes to himself affect his motivation to change and also how the behaviour of others towards him may have a positive or negative effect on his self-esteem.

Mary possibly needs the therapist to attempt to understand the problem from her point of view and explore the world as Mary sees it. A client-centred approach will provide the setting for the therapist to be empathetic to Mary's understanding of her voice problems and the reasons for these. Mary's inability to maintain the change which occurred during the last therapy will need to be explored non-judgementally and any ideas for maintaining voice quality in the future will need to grow out of Mary's own understanding of her behavioural patterns. Some of the exploratory approaches from Personal Construct Theory might well help both Mary and the therapist to understand why change seemed so hard to maintain.

*Knowledge*

For each of these clients the therapist will need to make sure his or her knowledge base is secure. Speech and language disorders related to cerebral palsy are diverse. The amount of brain damage, the presence or absence of concurrent sensory loss, the level of ability of the child, the child's personality, the child's life experiences and other unknown qualities that make one child different from another all have an effect. Specific language impairment can range from mild to severe, can coincide with many other learning difficulties or be very discrete, can range from phonological through grammatical to semantic-pragmatic problems or combinations of all three. Again, general ability, life experience and family situation can all have a major effect on the nature and outcomes of the problem. Voice disorders can be generated by medical conditions, by life experiences and by client personality. A sound knowledge of what may cause or exacerbate voice difficulties is essential.

Therapy is designed to bring about change. How an individual may respond to demands for change and how he or she may react to change as it is occurring is important knowledge for the therapist. Prochaska and DiClemente's model of change (1986), mentioned in Chapter 1, is an excellent discussion of the way in which change is facilitated or prevented by the level of awareness of the individual. An understanding of the processes that make change painful can be reached through a study of the 'constructs of transition', which define what happens to an individual when he or she is put under pressure to change or to look at him or herself differently, i.e. the individual is moving, or in transition, from one state of being to another (Dalton and Dunnet, 1992).

*Skills*

For each of these clients, the assessment and therapy approaches will be different. But what are the similarities? What skills that the clinician brings can be transferred from one to another?

1. Careful gathering of data is needed for each of these clients. No matter how different their presenting language problems, the clinician must be able to record, transcribe and analyse the linguistic problem.
2. Thoughtful planning, which can act as a blueprint for focusing the assessment or therapeutic endeavour, is needed. Writing a plan of assessment and therapy, conducting that assessment and undertaking therapy can be seen as skills that the therapist has had to learn by reading, thinking, watching and practising the activities.
3. Constant questioning of the information is an essential requirement. The therapist must engage in problem solving, analytical thinking and creative theorizing, and must be constantly querying what she is doing and where it is leading – 'Why is this as it is?', 'What does this mean?', 'Where does this behaviour stem from?', 'Who is important in this decision?'

**Imran**

*Assessment*

Assessment of Imran's difficulties took place within a multidisciplinary framework at the school. The professionals worked together in the nursery and all could keep an eye on Imran's behaviour in an informal setting. The nursery teacher, the physiotherapist, the occupational therapist and the speech and language therapist were the first to be involved. Imran had been diagnosed as having spastic cerebral palsy by a paediatrician prior to his being enrolled in the school and the team was interested in:

- the extent of the muscle involvement (the impairment)
- the effect of this on his mobility, language and ability to learn (the disability)
- the amount of problem this caused him and his family in everyday life (the handicap).

*Therapy*

Therapy took place alongside assessment – the two were interwoven. As soon as an area was assessed as needing input, this was addressed alongside continuing assessment of this and other areas. The speech and language therapist visited the school twice a week. She had a big caseload, as most of the children at the school needed assessment and many needed therapy of some kind. Intervention was therefore through non-intensive, individual or group direct therapy, as well as indirect therapy via the school staff and parents, who were encouraged to come into the school. The school had a policy of encouraging parental help with aspects of the learning process as well as offering a support group, run by the social worker, and a series of outings and events run by the parent-teacher association.

Prior to beginning work with Imran, the therapist had the following thoughts:

> For Imran, being in school with all these unknown people will probably be a shock as he has been only with his family up till now. He will also be exposed to a language that is unfamiliar to him. The paediatrician has suggested that he has a fairly severe spasticity, so all in all he will be a confused little boy. We must go slowly with the assessment and not push him too hard to start with. He may not have had much exposure to play with the sort of toys we have here. It is quite likely that he has only watched his cousins and siblings playing and has not really had a chance to play on his own. Toys, books and pictures will probably be unfamiliar to him.

The therapist then considered aims and objectives for the first six weeks of the school term. This was a common approach for all children and the objectives were written in to their individual education plans alongside those of the other professionals in the school.

### Short-term aims

1. To identify the nature of Imran's communication strengths and weaknesses.
2. To assess the level of spastic dysarthria.
3. To consider the need for augmentative communication devices.
4. To assess Imran's feeding abilities.

### Objectives

1. That Imran will have been observed in a number of communication situations and his behaviour will have been systematically recorded:
   * in contact with other children
   * in contact with the nursery teacher
   * in contact with other staff (e.g. in the dining room, with the physio-therapist in the swimming pool)
   * in contact with his mother
   * in contact with his brother and sister.
2. That Imran will have been encouraged to imitate as many tongue, lip and jaw movements as possible and records of the strength, accuracy and speed of these movements will be kept.
3. That Imran will be monitored for and encouraged to produce voice and his ability to control pitch and intensity and to sustain the voice will be recorded.
4. That Imran's ability to make his needs known through both verbal and non-verbal means will be recorded and his preferred mode of communication will be identified.

5. Imran will be observed during eating and drinking and his ability to chew and swallow will be recorded. This will take place alongside the occupational therapist's assessment of his ability to feed himself and his interest in foods, flavours, etc.

## David

### *Assessment*

During the initial interview with David and his mother it became clear that he had had difficulties with his language development from an early age. Unfortunately, the nature of his father's occupation had led to the family moving regularly and the language difficulty had not been dealt with when David was young. David's mother expressed anger that her regular concerns about his language development had been dismissed by a number of professionals through the years and he had only just been identified as having a problem at 13. She described a pattern of slow but regular development of both his sound system and his grammatical system. At the time he started school, he was intelligible but still behind. However, he tended to be a quiet child and was not picked up as a problem by the teachers. He was slow to develop reading skills, but had now been identified as somewhat slow in many areas (motor skills, maths and social skills). So again, the possibility of an underlying language problem was overlooked (though we know that reading and spelling problems are closely linked with persistent speech and language difficulties; Snowling and Stackhouse, 1996). David was a reticent boy who found it difficult to converse. He had an interest in motor bikes, which he seemed to be more at ease talking about, but even here he had to be prompted and questioned. He was dysfluent in discussion. He made numerous false starts, interjections and repetitions of single sounds and at times it was hard to follow what he was saying.

The therapist agreed to see him for a thorough investigation of his language problems and to offer David and his mother some strategies for dealing with the problems at this stage. It was necessary to contact his school, so that everyone could be clear about his difficulties and a combined approach could be instigated. The first session continued the process of understanding David's complex difficulties. Word-finding tasks presented little difficulty with easier words but more problems with more complex vocabulary. A phonological cue was immediately useful, suggesting that David had the vocabulary within his existing lexical memory but had difficulty retrieving the phonological make-up of words. He also had some problems with production of multisyllable words, where he omitted or transposed sounds. This suggested some motor planning problems. Imitation of these words was easy for him. However, imitation of long and grammatically complex sentences was very poor – David often lost the thread of these before getting to the end of them.

This was suggestive of auditory memory difficulties. Between this and the next session, the speech and language therapist had the following thoughts:

> David is a boy with complex difficulties. A way of thinking about his problems, and what is causing or caused by what, is necessary. If I put what I know about him on to a psycholinguistic framework such as that of Levelt (1989), I might better understand him and also what I might need to investigate and what might be best to suggest to teachers. I don't think he is a 'stutterer' though he is certainly dysfluent. His lack of friends is a worry and suggests that his unwillingness to talk does not just extend to adults. It seems important to build up his confidence and self-esteem. His mother's worry also needs to be addressed as this probably affects him too.

Following these thoughts, the therapist developed these aims and objectives for working with David.

### Aims

1. To assess David's level of difficulty in a range of cognitive and language areas such as:
   * comprehension of vocabulary and grammar
   * awareness of rhyme and of syllable structure
   * auditory memory.
2. To attempt to understand David's language and literacy problems from his own point of view.
3. To liaise with school and home in an endeavour for all to come to a common acceptance of the best approach to deal with David's problems.

### Objectives

1. That David will complete a range of formal and informal assessments in order for us to understand his language and reading problems more fully.
2. That David will be engaged in the process by undertaking ratings and being involved in discussion of his difficulties and in deciding how to approach changes.
3. To discuss fully David's academic difficulties with his teacher and to work out a joint programme that can be useful to both his language and his reading and writing problems.

### Mary

Following Mary's attendance at the three-monthly review, the speech and language therapist sat down to consider Mary's case. Her thoughts ran something like this:

Mary is an intelligent and capable adult who has found it difficult for some reason to maintain the skills she learned in her last sessions with me. Is this because something has changed or that the skills were not securely learned and therefore were susceptible to breakdown? It will be important to understand what has happened from Mary's point of view and not to bring my own assumptions into play. I would hope that, through providing a secure setting where Mary can explore the reasons for the return of her voice problems, I can give Mary the support she needs to regain the lost voice skills and to find a way of establishing them securely enough that they will maintain better in the future.

The therapist then wrote the following aims and objectives for Mary.

*Aims*

1. To explore Mary's attitudes to her voice and to voice change.
2. To ensure that Mary has a clear idea of the tasks and exercises that will reduce vocal abuse.
3. To encourage Mary to find ways of maintaining vocal change.

*Objectives*

1. That Mary will be clear about her own ability to change and blocks to changing, and that she will be able to identify these.
2. That Mary will have practised the voice techniques and shown her knowledge and competence in using them.
3. That Mary will have discussed some reasons why the changes that occurred in the previous therapy were not maintained and what she might do to enhance maintenance.

The aims and objectives presented here for the three clients can be seen as short-term, in that they are achievable within a reasonable time span. They will be part of a more global view that the therapist will have of the long-term outcomes for these clients. The long-term aims will be affected by the nature of the impairment, the degree of the disability and the quantity and quality of the handicap which arises from the problem. Imran has an impairment that will be with him for life. But the amount of disability is as yet unknown. How he and his family will adjust and cope with his physical handicap will be very important in his overall life achievements. David, too, has a pervasive disorder related to a less clear-cut impairment. His academic achievement is being affected by his problems and this is the area that needs to be addressed if he is not to be handicapped in his later years. Mary has a problem that could potentially handicap her chances in her chosen career. She has the potential to reduce vocal abuse and achieve a good level of vocal control. Her long-term outcomes are dependent on her managing the life stressors that affect this control.

**Plans and outcomes**

For each of these clients, a session plan and its outcomes will be presented as an example of how the short-term aims and objectives are converted into a plan for the day.

**Imran**

Look back at the aims and objectives for this series of six sessions. So far the therapist has recorded Imran's behaviour using the Preverbal Assessment-Intervention Profile (Connard, 1984) to get an idea of his visual and auditory awareness and his motor ability. Imran has proved difficult to assess because of a fairly severe level of spastic cerebral palsy. He shows no inclination to imitate articulatory movements. His responses to having his name called are erratic, but he shows interest in other people, both adults and children. The therapist has visited his home once with the bilingual co-worker. Imran spent his time in the family living room watching the other children at play. They would often take him things and show him objects and he would smile, then they would carry on with their game. His mother (Mrs A) was very busy with all the children but had a lot of support from her cousin. They took turns at feeding Imran, mostly in a near supine position. The family did not expect Imran to improve and seemed to accept him as he was, and as long as he was happy and well cared for they did not see that more should be done for him. At school Imran has proved to have some lip closure on to a spoon during feeding, but will not tolerate any lumps in his mouth. He shows an ability to push these forward with his tongue. His swallowing reflex is slow, but good once it is begun. This appears to be because Imran has difficulty moving the food back in his mouth.

Before planning the final session for a review meeting to discuss Imran, the therapist has the following thoughts:

> Imran seems very alert. He obviously recalls events and is enjoying the rhymes, songs and activities with the other children. He appears to be attempting to imitate some of the actions with the rhymes, such as moving his body forward and his head down when we sing 'all fall down'. He still needs quite a bit of physical support in order to participate in this way. Otherwise his head will fall forward and he will find it difficult to raise again. He does not like to be pushed though, and will wail and cry if anyone tries to make him do something when he doesn't want to. At home, demands are not made of him at all and this could be a problem in the long run. We must try to bring Mrs A into school as much as possible – but this is difficult because of her lack of English and her ability to travel (she can only come when her cousin's husband, who is a taxi driver, can bring them). The difference between our hopes and expectations for Imran and those of his family seems great at the moment. I must talk more to the bilingual assistant at the clinic to understand what the family might be thinking and wanting for Imran. In the meantime, he seems to be enjoying the activities with the other children in the nursery and it now seems to be the right time to assess his early potential for a communication board of some kind.

*Session 6*

*Aims*

1. To assess Imran's ability to vocalize on command.
2. To obtain information about his object to picture matching ability as a precursor to considering a basic communication board.
3. To assess whether Imran will make a deliberate choice.

*Objectives*

1. That Imran will make a vocal sound to activate a toy and that he will do this at least three out of five times.
2. That Imran will participate in and show ability to match during the object-picture game. He will need to show that he can do this consistently (four out of the five pictures).
3. That Imran will make a definite eye-pointing choice between banana and biscuit at drinks time.

*Procedures*

All activities will take place in the group as Imran definitely responds best when other children are involved. He does not respond well in a one-to-one session with an adult.

1. Introduce the monkey and the dog, both of which respond to sound. Encourage the children to all make noise to help them see the link and then give them individual turns to try and activate the toys.
2. Use the big pictures and matching toys. Ask the children to identify if their picture matches the toy that is being held up. Imran to look from toy to his picture if it matches.
3. Ask the nursery assistant to hold a banana and a biscuit up to Imran and wait till he eye-points, then give him his choice. Observe and record.

*Methods*

1. In a group of five children all seated in circle (with the occupational therapist and assistant), encourage a lot of vocalization – you may need to warm the children up with a physical rolling game first (short session with physiotherapist prior to this?). Introduce monkey and dog, tell a story about them sleeping and being woken up by noises. Give all the children turns (at least five each).
2. As Imran seems to have better head control when in his standing frame, stand the children around the table and place a picture in front of each child. Hold up a toy and ask for the child who has the picture to indicate by vocalizing, eye-pointing, etc. Again, each child must have at least five tries.
3. Have chart ready for drink and biscuit time.

*Evaluation and outcomes*

1. Imran got very excited about the monkey and dog and it was difficult for him to stop vocalizing. While he tended to start and stop alongside the other children, when he was asked to have a turn, he only once seemed to manage to deliberately vocalize. So it seems at present that vocalization is not under his voluntary control.
2. Imran was quite able when it came to the matching (this is something that has been concentrated on in the nursery). He definitely showed excitement when his picture matched the toy. He found it less easy to eye-point to his picture – he did this two out of the five times. Unfortunately, he also became excited when other children had a match – though he did not seem to move his arm around as much (need to check this out further).
3. During drink and biscuit time, he first seemed to be choosing only the item on his left but, once he had been given the banana, which he didn't like, he began to make deliberate efforts to choose the biscuit. He did this on four consecutive occasions.

*Outcomes over the 6-week period*

Looking back at the aims and objectives for the six-week period the speech and language therapists can comment on the following:

1. Imran's communicative strengths and weaknesses. He definitely prefers to be with the other children. He also responds to his little brother of 3, who has come in once with his mother and aunt. He seems more cautious of adults, except for his mother. He shows his interest by smiling, vocalizing, waving his left arm and deliberately touching (in his case it is hitting because he can't control the extent of the movement) the child next to him. He will give fleeting eye contact, but this is more difficult for him.
2. Imran appears to have a severe spastic dysarthria. He has little control over vocalization though he has shown he can start and stop his voice with the other children. His lip closure is fairly good and he does not drool excessively unless sucking on some food. Tongue movements are limited to some slight forwards and backwards spontaneous movement during feeding.
3. Imran has definite needs, which he makes known through laughing and crying. He is also capable of deliberately choosing by turning his head and eyes towards the chosen object. He seems to be beginning to recognize a picture-object match. So it is possible that a picture communication board of some kind might be something to work towards as he becomes more capable of making deliberate actions.
4. Imran has a good swallow reflex but his ability to bite and chew is poor. He needs to be gradually introduced to more solids and this needs to

be done alongside a programme of encouraging his family to experiment more with foods for him.

### Conclusions

It is clear that the speech and language therapist achieved her aims and objectives over the six-week period. These aims were cautious – they looked only a short step ahead. They took into account the fact that this child has severe difficulties and long-term outcomes will be dependent on his developing motor control, his cognitive abilities, which are still little known, and his developing ability to understand English. He has pervasive and long-term difficulties and as yet his potential is unknown.

But the process of assessing and offering help to Imran has begun. The extent of his difficulties is becoming known. All members of the multidisciplinary team are contributing to an understanding of his needs. His family is being included, and education and support are being offered. Imran's speech and language development will proceed hand in hand with his growing motor control and cognitive abilities. The speech and language therapist can only provide the encouragement, materials and information for others that will enhance this development; she cannot accelerate his maturation or expect more than he is neurologically capable of achieving at this point in time.

## David

### Session 2

Prior to this session, the therapist hypothesized that David seemed to have a problem with the phonological representation of words and with motor planning. He had had difficulty in discussing his own thoughts and feelings, which led the therapist to decide on a technique from brief therapy known as the 'miracle question'. This required David to think about what would happen if he woke up one morning without this problem: what would change, what would he be like (Selekman, 1993)? Both David and his mother were to separately write down some ideas around this thought during the week.

### Aims

1. To continue to assess David's phonological and motor skills.
2. To discuss the 'miracle question' task and the implications of what both David and his mother have written about what may change.
3. To obtain a sample of David's spontaneous language for analysis of his fluency and grammatical skills.
4. To discuss with David the forthcoming visit to school.

## Objectives

1. That David will complete the rhyming tasks and the Spoonerism and tongue-twister tasks from the Phonological Battery Assessment (Frederickson et al., 1997) and will discuss these with the clinician.
2. That David will discuss the miracle question, his responses to it and the reason why he said what he did in relation to it.
3. That David's mother will also have a chance to reflect on her own responses to this task.
4. That David will talk about his main interest – motor bikes – for some while (he has been asked to bring in his motor bike magazine) and a tape and video recording will be done of him for analysis.
5. That David will have understood the reason for the therapist's visit to school and the areas that will be discussed with the therapist will be explained to him.

## Procedures

1. Draw David a picture of the language-processing mechanism and show him what levels we are trying to find out about.
2. Complete the rhyming, Spoonerism and tongue-twister tasks.
3. Use the miracle question sequence, scaling questions and coping sequence from Selekman (1993:63-70) to talk David through his feelings about his school difficulties. Do the same with David's mother. This can be done together or separately depending on the wishes of both of them.
4. Make sure the consent form for video and audio taping has been signed. Set up the recording and ask David to talk about motor bikes. Do not use too many direct questions, use prompts, queries and comments to encourage him to keep talking.

## Evaluation and outcomes

1. David was interested in the psycholinguistic model and became quite enthusiastic about identifying the levels where he had most difficulty and those he found easy.
2. Within this framework of being scientists and exploring issues about ourselves (Kelly, 1963), David was very motivated to try out the rhyme judgement and motor tasks. He was able to judge rhymes from pictures of well-known and relatively simple words but had more difficulty when the words were longer and less frequent such as 'excavate' and 'eliminate'. This was in part due to his difficulty in retrieving the vocabulary and partly because he may have had problems generating a phonological image of these words. When they were written down, he had no problems identifying the rhyme. He found it difficult to

produce some of the Spoonerisms but not others. So he easily gave 'dig bog' for 'big dog' but could not manage a sound swap for 'Reginald Pickering'. This was possibly due to short-term memory problems – he seemed unable to hold this name in his head in order to manipulate the phonemes. Tongue twisters were very difficult for him. He definitely appears to have problems with complex sequences of sounds, and when he tried to speed up, he became completely lost.

3. Discussion of the 'miracle question' was very useful. David and his mother chose to discuss it together – in fact they had begun this process at home. It was evident that David sees an improvement in his reading and writing as being of use to him in making friends, while his mother is more concerned about his long-term academic prospects. The use of 'coping' questions focused both of them more on to what David had achieved so far, how he had managed to deal with school for all these years and who he identified as being friends or possible friends. David and his mother agreed to think about David's social activities and what might help him gain more friends.

4. David had an enormous amount of knowledge and information about motor bikes and was very keen to discuss this. A good recording was made. During this discussion, it was felt that he was mainly dysfluent when he was trying to plan how to say something. He often changed track in the middle of a sentence and sometimes did this so often that the therapist lost the meaning of what he was saying. It was suggested that he write about motor bikes for next session in order for further assessment of his writing skills to be made.

5. David was informed that the therapist was due to visit his teacher during this week. He seemed unconcerned about this.

*Outcomes over the 4-week assessment period*

1   Assessment of cognitive and language difficulties had led to the following information on David:
   • comprehension of vocabulary and grammar on the low end of the normal range
   • some complex grammatical structures difficult due to short-term memory problems
   • auditory memory seems to be a main problem for David
   • complex motor sequences difficult
   • planning and executing longer utterances problematic due to the above difficulties.

2   Exploration of David's own perceptions and feelings has proved useful and the following changes have already occurred:
   • David and his mother are talking about and exploring his school difficulties together
   • David has joined a motor bike enthusiasts' website and is quite excited about communicating in this way.

3 Joint programmes between school, therapist and home have been initi-
ated. While David's complex difficulties are unlikely to show sudden or
quick change, all parties are sharing information and are confident that
change is possible. The ongoing planning and preparation of
programmes for David will be a joint responsibility between the therapist and his teacher. Additional help is being sought by the school from
the Special Services Division, which offers support for specific
academic problems encountered by pupils.

*Conclusions*

Again, the short-term aims and objectives were achieved for David. The
process of change, which is what therapy is about, had definitely begun
and all parties involved were actively engaged in working towards a
positive outcome. For David, the process of improving his academic skills
had not yet started, and the outcomes of this were as yet unknown.
However, David's strengths had been acknowledged, paths of communication had been opened up and attempts were being made to understand
the reasons for his difficulties.

Measuring these outcomes in relation to the model of impairment,
disability, handicap and distress on a six-point scale would result in the
changes shown in Table 4.1.

Table 4.1: Change in David over four-week assessment period

| Domain | 1 very poor | 2 | 3 | 4 | 5 | 6 no problem |
|---|---|---|---|---|---|---|
| **Impairment** understanding of problem by all | | * | | + | | full awareness |
| **Disability** improvement in reading and writing | | * | + | | | |
| **Handicap** making friends | | * | + | | | |
| **Distress** feelings of worth | * | | + | | | |

* indicates first completion at initial interview.
+ indicates completion after 4 weeks.

**Mary**

*Session 1*

*Aims*

1. To revise the procedures we had explored in the last series of
   sessions.

2. To discuss with Mary the situation now and why she feels her voice has deteriorated.

*Objectives*

1. That Mary will have satisfactorily demonstrated:
   • gentle onsets
   • postural awareness
   • breathing techniques previously taught.
2. That Mary will have had an opportunity to explore reasons for the lack of maintenance of voice change.

*Procedures*

1. Ask Mary to define the factors in her life that are the same and different now to those during the past sessions.
2. Use rating scales to define the level of:
   • voice use
   • shouting during the day
   • general levels of stress.
3. To discuss with Mary any changes in her routines in terms of teaching or other aspects of daily life.
4. Ask Mary to demonstrate:
   • diaphragmatic breathing
   • breathy/not hard attack onsets
   • control of pitch and loudness.
5. Observe the level of tension in neck and shoulders – ask Mary about relaxation exercises.

*Evaluation and outcomes*

Mary was keen to talk and had to be reminded to take breaths and not talk 'on the ends of her breath'. She described her school situation as being different now because of a new head who was very organized and demanded that his staff have written records of everything they did. This meant that Mary was working long hours in the evening to detail information that had previously been taken for granted. She was feeling very demoralized by this and was questioning her own ability as a teacher. She commented that her pupils had always done well in the various assessments set them so she didn't know why it was necessary to do all this extra paperwork. The additional time spent doing this made her feel guilty about loss of time with her own children – two boys of 8 and 10.

Mary spent most of the session talking about these feelings – it did not seem appropriate to do the ratings, so these were dropped. However, it was evident that, as she talked, she built up excessive tension in her shoulders and took less deep breaths. Towards the end of the session the therapist reminded her that it was important to review her skills in voice control. When she was thinking of them, she was able to breathe well, to control the outflow of breath and to keep her onsets relaxed and soft.

It was agreed that Mary needed to consider how her life was being driven by the need to complete the school paperwork and whether anything could be done about this. She was to think about her techniques to improve her voice and see where she should apply them. She was to take 15 minutes each day to do her relaxation exercises.

After this session the speech and language therapist discussed Mary with a colleague and the discussion went something like this:

> I wonder if Mary is being realistic about what is expected of her from school or whether she has misconstrued the head teacher's requests for more paper work? It is obvious that Mary is aware of and able to use the techniques learned but it appears that that she is not putting this into practice during her school day. This may be as a result of the pressure she is feeling from the head teacher. It seems important for Mary to be clear about what her week consists of, to reduce her workload outside of school hours and to give herself more time to relax and think about her voice. This seems to be the area that needs to be focused on in therapy. Possibly a self-characterization (Fransella and Dalton, 1990) written by Mary relating to herself as she feels she is now versus herself as she would wish to be might start her thinking about what she would like to and be able to change.

The therapist had originally offered Mary four sessions to re-evaluate her ability to change her voice and to consider why she had been unable to maintain the previous changes. Mary attended for two further sessions and then decided that she was sufficiently confident that she needed no further input from the therapist. Evaluation of the third session revealed the following:

- After writing a self-characterization, Mary had discussed her situation with the head teacher and realized that she had obviously misunderstood his request. He had expressed concern about her voice and reflected on her need to be careful with it. He had had experience with other teachers who had suffered from voice loss and was sympathetic to the problem. All this made Mary feel more confident and less overwhelmed by her problem. She said that discussing it with him had made her feel that she no longer had to hide the fact that she was having voice problems.
- Mary had not completed a chart of her relaxation. She said she had not done much of this because she felt so good after talking to the head that she did not feel she needed it. We discussed the fact that she will not always feel so good and looked at the stages of change and what can bring about relapse. Mary seemed a bit resistant to this – she did not appear to want to think about relapse. However, Mary said that she had started a yoga class where she knew she would be encouraged to

relax regularly. She felt she would be better at doing this in a group than on her own.

- Mary said she was happy with the changes she had made and felt in control of her life and her voice at this time. It was pointed out that regular practice of the techniques she had learned was very important. It was agreed that therapy would be discontinued and a further review would take place after three months. If she still felt positive at this stage, she would be discharged.

## Conclusions

The conclusions following this period of therapy with Mary will be written in the form of a report to her consultant ENT specialist (see Figure 4.5).

---

Dear Dr Smith

re:     Mary T 2.5.63
        24 East Speed Street
        Honeywell
        CN4 3BT

Mary T returned for a series of three voice therapy sessions from 3.7.97 to 17.7.97.

She presented with a history of voice loss at the end of the school day and some feelings of irritation in her throat.

Therapy consisted of looking at issues in her school life which may have exacerbated the problem and revising previously learned techniques for voice control and vocal hygiene.

Mary quickly demonstrated that she could recall the techniques. However, she did not use them regularly. Her vocal hygiene was, on the whole, good and she needed few reminders to avoid certain irritants. The main factor seemed to be her adjustment at school to the demands of a new headteacher. During the three sessions, she was able to discuss her situation with her head and thus reduce the underlying tensions that had developed.

I have agreed to see Mary again in three months' time as I have some concerns that she may find maintenance of the improved voice difficult. At that time, if she has continued to use the preferred breath control and relaxation methods, I shall discharge her from my care.

I shall keep you informed of the situation.

Yours sincerely

Sandra Black BSc, Reg MRCSLT
Speech and Language Therapist

---

**Figure 4.5:** Letter to Mary's referral agent.

**General conclusions**

The information presented on these three clients will hopefully have made explicit some of the important issues originally raised about the reality of being a therapist. The therapist with each client was operating from a particular philosophical base. The underlying theories touched on were drawn from:

- client-centred therapy
- brief therapy
- personal construct therapy
- family therapy
- learning theory
- operant conditioning
- cognitive therapy.

Overall, the therapist was operating from a humanistic perspective, believing that the client was capable of being able in some way to direct his or her life choices.

The knowledge that the therapist called on to actually conduct the sessions was based on an understanding of:

- language acquisition and development
- bilingualism and its effect on language
- muscle control difficulties in cerebral palsy
- reinforcement schedules
- psycholinguistic models of language reception and expression
- auditory processing
- memory and language
- understanding of the vocal mechanism
- reciprocal inhibition.

The therapist found the model of change suggested by Prochaska and DiClemente (1986) to be invaluable in helping her to make decisions about:

- where to start – at what stage of change is this individual (pre-contemplative, contemplative, active, maintaining)
- where to focus in therapy – what level is most appropriate (symptomatic, interpersonal, systems, intrapersonal)
- what processes are likely to change and what techniques might encourage this to occur (self re-evaluation, environmental re-evaluation, counterconditioning, stimulus control, environmental control, etc.).

The ideas the therapist came up with, as well as the ways of bringing the changes about, grew out of her knowledge and experience, and her willingness to talk to others and read around the issues. She was able to think creatively because she was secure that she was as knowledgeable as possible, that she could call upon others, that the clients were also involved in the decision making about their therapy, and that she and her clients were approaching the therapeutic situation with a hypothesis-generating and testing model. She therefore was confident that she understood both the process of and the practical aspects of therapy.

# Chapter 5
# Working with Other People

It is implicit that any clinical relationship involves working with others. During the past 20 years, however, there seems to have been an increase in the range of working relationships in which a speech and language clinician may be involved.

Although direct intervention with the client, either on an individual or group basis is central to their work, the clinician is likely to be involved in:

- working with relatives and carers
- working with and through other staff
- the training of carers and other workers.

## Working with families and carers

The relatives or people providing day-to-day care for the client are extremely important. They are likely to have the most amount of contact with them, and will shape and influence the environment in which they will communicate. They are therefore a great source of support that can be harnessed in the intervention process. At the same time, relatives and carers may have a high degree of emotional involvement with the client, and may also require support and assistance from the professionals involved. In order for them to provide appropriate support for the client, relatives must understand the nature of the client's difficulties and have realistic expectations for the future. As part of the initial assessment process you will be seeking the perceptions of the problem from the carers, how this impinges on the client's life and what are the expectations for change. It is important that the long-term and short-term aims of intervention are negotiated with the client and carers, and meet the client's needs in their particular family and social network.

### Parents

The Children Act 1989 reaffirmed the view of the government that children are best looked after within the family and the best way to help the child is by professionals working in partnership with parents. The Act introduced the concept of 'parental responsibility' to replace the previous notion of parental rights. Parental responsibility means that:

- children should not be viewed as the property of parents
- child rearing is primarily the responsibility of parents
- the role of the state is to assist parents with these responsibilities but not to interfere with family life.

It is now recognized that professionals should work in partnership with parents. Partnership can be defined as:

> A working relationship exists with shared sense of purpose, respect and willingness to negotiate. Partnership also implies that parents and workers share information, responsibility, skills, decision making, and accountability. (Houghton and McColgan, 1995: 99)

For the speech and language clinician working with children, this relationship with parents should be central to their organization of intervention. In the community clinic the parent may often be responsible for bringing the child to the clinic so that regular contact is established, and good working relationships may be easy to foster. During the assessment period the parent will be able to provide a wealth of information about the general development of the child. They will be able to give more specific information about the development of communication and the particular problems the child is encountering. The parent should also be closely involved in the decision-making process, and aims and objectives for intervention should be negotiated and agreed with them (and the child where this is appropriate). Parents will often be the main implementers of the intervention programme and should, wherever possible, be an integral part of the clinic session.

When the speech and language clinician makes recommendations for carry-over work to be continued at home, it is important that realistic and achievable demands are made on the parents. Suggestions need to take into account the home environment, the understanding and capabilities of the parents and the other demands made on their time by work and family life.

It is extremely valuable to observe and work with the child in the home environment, although unfortunately the policies of some speech and language departments discourage this, viewing it as excessively time consuming. However, observing the child in the home allows the clinician to:

- observe the child's communication skills in a naturalistic environment
- assess the demands made for communication within the home
- formulate an intervention plan which capitalizes on the environment, utilizes the resources of the home and fits into the family routine

- make a more realistic assessment of what can be expected in terms of home support
- encourage the parent to express their opinions in a familiar environment where they may feel more confident than in the clinic setting
- encourage the child and the family to see the intervention as part of the everyday context, thereby encouraging generalization and carry over.

There are a number of intervention programmes that have been developed to involve and empower the parents in the management of the child's communication problems. For example, the Hanen approach consists of a series of training sessions for groups of parents (Girolametto, 1988). Here they are encouraged to share their experiences with others in a similar position. The programme aims to influence their attitude to the child's difficulties, as well as teaching skills to facilitate language development.

Research by Sally Ward (1994) has shown that early intervention within the home can significantly improve the communication abilities of young children through relatively minimal involvement. The Willstar programme takes children from one year old and aims to improve listening skills. This work is carried out by parents in the home environment. Results have shown that this intervention has positive effects when compared to a non-treatment group.

In schools, this continued and active involvement of parents may be more difficult to foster. The clinician may not have contact with parents on a regular basis and may be working through teaching staff and assistants. However, it is important that parents are kept informed of what is happening with their child, and that they continue to be involved in the intervention process. This contact may be maintained by:

- writing in the home-school dairy (these are commonly used in special schools where children are transported to school by the education authority, so that parents may have little day-to-day contact with the school)
- arranging to see parents when they drop the child at school or collect them at the end of the day
- inviting parents in to the speech and language session
- being involved in parents evenings and other school activities
- arranging training sessions, coffee mornings, etc., for groups of parents
- regular contact by phone
- visiting the child at home in school holidays
- writing regular reports in accessible language
- attendance at annual review meetings.

### Children with significant special needs

For the parent of a child with significant and long-term difficulties there will inevitably be a period of anxiety and confusion as they come to terms with the situation. In the early stages they may experience a range of emotional and practical problems including:

- grieving for the 'loss' of the normal child they were expecting
- anxiety about short-term health issues
- embarrassment and anxiety about telling family and friends
- readjustment of plans to return to work, arrangements for child care, etc.
- concern about the child's long-term future
- confusion and lack of knowledge about the impact of the diagnosis and the long-term implications in terms of development, education, etc.

It is important that all professionals involved with the child and family are aware of how parents are feeling, and provide appropriate and timely support. Much confusion and anxiety can be caused when parents receive conflicting information from different people. It is important that you restrict your discussions to areas of direct relevance to speech and language. It is useful to establish contact with the other professionals involved with the child, so that you are aware of what other information the parents are being given.

It is recognized that stress and anxiety influences how people are able to process information. The same details and conversations may need to be repeated several times for understanding to take place and for the information to be assimilated.

It may also be useful to put parents in contact with suitable support groups, for example The Down's Syndrome Association, Scope, etc. Information about local groups should be readily available. For less common disorders the 'In Touch' organization provides invaluable information and aims to put parents in contact with other families experiencing similar difficulties. The Internet is also a useful place for information and contacts for parents and professionals (see useful addresses in Appendix).

In this discussion we have focused on the parents, but it is important to remember that other members of the family will be influenced by the situation. Brothers and sisters, grandparents, aunts and uncles, foster and respite parents, nannies and child minders, may all be involved in the care of the child and may be invaluable assistants in the intervention process. They may also need support and information to more fully understand the child's difficulties. However, it is important to remember the issue of confidentiality. Permission must be gained from parents before information is disclosed to other members of the family or other carers involved with the child.

### The older child or adolescent

As the child moves into the teenage years there will be a gradual change in their relationship with their parents. At this time the opinions and influence of their peers will take on greater significance. There is no legal age limit when a child can give permission for treatment. Judgement needs to be made on the child's ability to understand the implications of the decision. It may be the case that the parents are keen for intervention to continue, whereas the child does not see the value. A decision will need to be made as to whose opinion is the most important. However, if the child is not interested or is hostile to intervention, the potential for change is likely to be significantly reduced. It may be better to discontinue intervention, until such a time as the child seeks help for themselves. But coming to terms with this decision can be difficult for parents.

## The adult

With the older child or adult client there may be little or no involvement with other members of the family. Any discussion with a third party should only be with the permission of the client. However, the involvement of family and friends can be an extremely useful part of the intervention programme. It can provide a view of the client's day-to-day communication difficulties and their current lifestyle and communication needs.

### Adults with an acquired disorder

For the client with an acquired communication difficulty, their relatives and friends may be able to provide information about their level of communication and lifestyle prior to the trauma. They will also be able to discuss the demands currently being made upon the client and their present communication needs.

### Example

Mrs S is 85 years old, lives alone and has recently had a stroke resulting in severe mixed aphasia. You learn from her daughter that before her stroke, Mrs S spent much of her day reading books provided by the mobile library. She was unable to get out to the shops so provided her daughter with a weekly list of requirements. This information will influence the priority that needs to be given to reading and writing skills.

At the same time, the relatives are likely to be going through a period of readjustment as they came to terms with the changes that have occurred in their loved one. The communication problem may mean that the client can no longer be as involved in family discussion and decision making. Both they and members of the family may need support to adjust to their change in role.

The relatives and friends may also be a useful therapeutic agent and should, wherever possible, be involved in the intervention process. They may want to attend all therapy sessions or visit intermittently, or contact may be maintained through telephone or letter. However, all contact and discussion should be with the consent of the client. In some cases they may not wish to have their relatives involved.

In some instances the relatives may not want to attend clinic sessions. This may give them a brief respite from the demands of caring for the client. There may also be times when they may wish to talk to the clinician without the client being present. This may give them an opportunity to express feelings and ask questions that they would not do in front of the client.

This support to relatives should be an integral part of the intervention process. It should enable them to understand what has happened, the impact on the client's ability to communicate and ways that may help them to communicate effectively with the client. It may also be helpful for the clinician to arrange for relatives and friends to meet others in a similar position so that they can share experiences and discuss different ways of handling the situation.

### Adults with a non-acquired disorder

For adults who have had a life-long communication difficulty, there may be a period of adjustment as parents come to accept that their child is becoming an adult. There are likely to be a number of changes in roles and relationships, with the 'child' taking greater responsibility in the decision-making process. At this time, there may also be changes in the communication expectations and demands made upon them. These periods of transition from school to work and from family home to independent or sheltered accommodation can mean that existing communication abilities may be challenged. Families may have a well-established routine of communication where they have 'tuned into' the client's system. There may be a need to extend communication skills or provide some sort of augmentative system to facilitate communication with a broader range of people.

## Working with other professionals

This collaboration may be with individual colleagues employed by the same organization or those from other public sector agencies, such as education or social service departments, or the private and voluntary sector. Examples might include:

1. Health:
   - physiotherapists
   - nurses
   - health visitors
   - health care assistants
   - consultants
   - general practitioners
   - clinical psychologists.
2. Education
   - teachers
   - non-teaching assistants
   - educational psychologists.

3. Social welfare
   - social workers
   - staff in nurseries/family centres
   - staff in homes for aged people
   - staff in social education centres.
4. Voluntary
   - staff and volunteers engaged by the Stroke Association
   - staff and volunteers engaged by Invalid Children's Aid Nationwide (I–CAN)
   - staff and volunteers engaged by Association for All Speech Impaired Children
   - individual volunteers.
5. Private
   - staff in Nursing Homes
   - Independent Practitioners (employed by a public service agency).

This increasing move towards greater team and multidisciplinary working originally stemmed from examples of good practice developed to provide effective and coordinated client management. There is evidence that such an approach can enhance client care. For example, Pennington and Windett (1994) demonstrated that a team approach to alternative and augmentative communication (AAC) had benefits for both staff and target children. There was also less duplication of services and more relevant application of the skills and knowledge of the professionals involved. Wilson and Laidler (1990) report a significant change in the length of stay for patients on rehabilitation wards following the development of a multi-disciplinary approach to patient care.

As well as these benefits for the clients there are also advantages for the staff involved. Collaborative practice in the UK has also been endorsed by the formalization and official recognition of a number of teams. For example:

- *The Child Protection Team*. A team usually comprising representatives from education, health and social welfare agencies, as well as the police and voluntary agencies. This team is responsible for the coordinated investigation of suspected child abuse, the maintenance of the local Child Protection Register and the development of appropriate policies and procedures dealing with child protection.
- *Learning Disability Team*. A team frequently based within a social service department, providing a multidisciplinary assessment, support and advisory service for people with learning disabilities and their families. This team usually includes a community nurse and social worker, and may also involve physiotherapists, occupational therapists, speech and language clinicians and clinical psychologists.
- *Rehabilitation Team*. A team usually based in a rehabilitation unit of a hospital. It may be led by a rehabilitation consultant, but will include

support from a range of therapy services, a psychologist, nursing and social welfare staff. The aim of the team will be to provide a coordinated package of rehabilitation and support for clients referred to them.

There has also been increasing reference to the importance of collaborative practice in a range of government guidelines and legislation. The need for multidisciplinary collaboration has been highlighted in relation to:

- Child care: UK, *Children Act 1989* stresses the need for a coordinated response to child care and protection, and the development of clear communication between professionals.
- Education: USA, *Education for All Handicapped Children Act 1975*; UK, *Code of Practice 1993* emphasizes the need for a team approach to the assessment and support of children with special educational needs; UK, 1997 DFEE Green Paper *Excellence for all children: meeting special educational needs* states that there will be improved cooperation between LEAs, social service departments and health authorities by the year 2002.
- Health care: UK, *The Health of the Nation 1992* discusses the need for the development of good working relationships between various staff groups.
- Community care: UK, *The NHS and Community Care Act 1990* called for the development of clear policies between health and social welfare agencies to cater for the support of clients within their community.

Further, at an international level the World Health Organization's targets for the *Health For All by the Year 2000* stresses the importance of an holistic approach to health and disease. This stresses the need for cross-professional education and training, and hence promotes collaborative practice.

## Terminology

Before examining some of the issues that need to be considered when working in a team setting, it is important to be clear about the terminology used. This is given in Table 5.1, and it will be useful to consider each of these terms in a little more detail.

### Collaboration

Any example of working together could be described as collaboration. In this context the term is used to describe informal relationships which would not justify the title of 'team'. The speech and language clinician may collaborate with a colleague when they plan a language group together, or collaborate with a health visitor or GP when concerned about the needs of a particular child in their care. Frequently these relationships are short-lived and client- or problem-focused. The skills of clear communication and mutual respect for each other's professional expertise and personal opinion are vital, and these informal links, if managed successfully, may lead to more frequent and longer-term professional relationships.

**Table 5.1**: Definitions

---

### DEFINITIONS

---

**Collaboration**: to work jointly together

**Group**: a number of persons located close together, or classed together

**Teamwork**: work done by several associates with each doing a part, but all subordinating personal prominence to the efficiency of the whole

**Unidisciplinary**: working with colleagues from one's own field

**Multidisciplinary**: a team comprising members of a range of different professionals, which does not necessarily share working practices or common aims

**Interdisciplinary**: working with other disciplines in the development of jointly planned objectives/programmes

**Transdisciplinary**: committed to teaching, learning and working with others across traditional discipline boundaries, this is likely to involve the transference of information and skills traditionally associated with one discipline to team members from other disciplines

**Inter-agency**: working with other disciplines employed by agencies different from our own, this can involve interdisciplinary, multidisciplinary or transdisciplinary collaboration.

---

### Groups and teamwork

The terms 'group' and 'team' are often used interchangeably. However, there is an important distinction between them. People may be 'grouped' together for a whole range of different reasons, but they may not work together in any meaningful or effective way. Often it is hoped that what may start out as a 'group' will develop into an effective team that will share skills and knowledge for the benefit of other team members and the clients whom they serve. However, the development of an effective team will involve both time and effort. There has been a considerable amount of research into group and team formation. The most important factors appear to be:

- group/team development
- roles within the team

- leadership style
- decision-making strategies
- purpose and tasks
- conflict resolution.

## Group/team development

It is now commonly accepted that the group goes through a number of recognizable stages from formation to becoming an effective working unit, or team. Tuckman (1965) suggests that there are at least four important stages to group development:

1. Forming. At this initial stage, group members are likely to feel unsure and will be concerned with testing out the boundaries of appropriate and expected behaviour. At this stage the group members may be heavily reliant on the group leader for guidance.
2. Storming. As group members become more familiar with each other, conflict may arise. Issues of status, prestige and power may need to be resolved. Members may feel a need to assert and clarify their own role and sphere of influence within the group. It is believed that if this period of conflict is not experienced during the early stages of group development, the group may be operating with unresolved conflict and poorly defined boundaries. This may create difficulties later on.
3. Norming. Gradually as conflicts are resolved and issues of boundaries and attitudes are clarified, the group may be able to compromise and develop a set of shared attitudes and values. At the same time more clearly defined role expectations, division of labour and established norms of behaviour may emerge.
4. Performing. It is only at this stage that the team members can focus on getting on with the tasks in hand. Hopefully, good communication channels have been established and the team has a sense of shared goals and responsibility.

A fifth stage could be added to this process:

5. Reforming. Even an effective group may not be continually harmonious. Changes in group membership, the need to meet critical deadlines, external pressures and changes in expectations may lead the group into another period of uncertainty. At this stage it may be necessary for the group to recycle back through earlier phases of development.

## Roles within the team

It is important that the clinician is clear about their own role and contribution in any working relationship. Are they coming together as equals, with equal responsibility for decision making, or is it a relationship of manager and subordinate, mentor and apprentice or student and supervisor?

Frequently we may fail to negotiate and clarify the issues of expectations and responsibility that may lead to misunderstanding, reduplication or neglect of important tasks, poor communication and eventual breakdown in relationships. Bower (1987) identifies a number of issues that may lead to stress and burn out for advisory special needs teachers. These factors may also be significant for other professionals working in an advisory capacity.

- Role expectation conflict: stress is generated as a result of a mismatch between a person's own expectation of a role and the expectations which others have of the same role. For example, this may occur in a school setting where the speech and language clinician and the teacher may have differing expectations of the role that they each play in relation to a child with a specific language disorder.
- Self-role conflict: stress can be generated when there is a gap between the way people see themselves and the way they are required to behave. Often the professional may have a clear view of how they would like their role to develop. This may be in conflict with the practical implementation in a particular setting.
- Role isolation: stress occurs when the individual feels that those occupying other roles, and with whom she has to interact, are psychologically distant. This can be particularly difficult for the clinician who spends little time in one location and has little contact with other professionals from a similar background. In this situation the development of supportive relationships can be problematic.
- Role erosion: stress is likely to be experienced in an organization that is redefining or creating new roles. This has been experienced by some speech and language professionals. For example, where the increase in involvement with clients with feeding and swallowing problems following a stroke, has led to less emphasis on their communication difficulties.
- Role ambiguity: stress may be caused when people are not clear about the expectations that others have of them, and results in low job satisfaction and low self-confidence. This can be a problem experienced by speech and language therapy students who may not feel confident to clarify their role with their clinical teacher. It is important that professionals discuss and negotiate with others about what are realistic expectations and how these can best be met.
- Role overload: stress occurs when there are too many or unrealistic expectations, even when they are clearly defined. This may be a quantitative or a qualitative overload. For the speech and language clinician it is important to be clear about what *can* be fulfilled, as well as stating what is not possible, so that overload can be avoided. This can be

particularly difficult for the clinician working in a number of settings where staff may be unaware of the expectations and demands of other areas of their work.

- Role inadequacy: stress may be created if the worker feels that she has insufficient skills or knowledge to adequately fulfil the role. This may be particularly true for the newly qualified clinician who may lack support and confidence. The opportunity to discuss this with a more experienced clinician may be vital. This may help to identify areas where additional training and professional development may be needed.
- Role stagnation: finally it should be remembered that as people 'grow into' their role, they may eventually risk becoming stale or fixed in their work. This may create particular tension if the task or composition of the team then changes (from Bower, 1987).

Good communication and negotiation may help to avoid some of the pitfalls, but it is important to regularly review working relationships so that unnecessary stress can be avoided. In any team context it is worth spending some time discussing the roles and expected contributions of team members. The following checklist may provide a useful starting point:

- What is the overall shared purpose of the team?
- What is each member aiming to do?
- What does this entail?
- Is the team supported by appropriate management to enable them to do this?
- Who is going to take responsibility for each aspect?
- Is there equal responsibility?
- Who takes overall responsibility?
- Is there equal commitment by all team members?

Considerable work on the definition of team roles has been carried out by Meredith Belbin (1993). He provides a useful questionnaire that can help team members to recognize their contribution to the group and may help the team to identify gaps in the 'team profile'. He defines the following roles that may operate in a group. Each role brings its own set of strengths and weaknesses, and it is the overall balance and combination of the team that results in success or failure. Interestingly the clinician may fulfil more than one role within a team, or take on different roles depending on the composition of the group, the task in hand and how they perceive their role within the particular team.

## Belbin's team roles

- Plant: this is the creative and imaginative member of the group who may come up with novel and unorthodox solutions to problems.

Weaknesses: may ignore details and is not always a good communicator.

- Resource investigator: an extrovert member of the group with good communication skills and enthusiasm, good at exploring opportunities and developing contacts. Weaknesses: may be overoptimistic and lose interest before the project is completed.
- Coordinator: this member may be good at chairing the discussion, has a skill in clarifying goals and promoting decision making, and is a good delegator. Weaknesses: may be manipulative and too willing to delegate.
- Shaper: this member thrives on pressure and has the drive and courage to overcome obstacles. Weaknesses: may provoke others and hurt people's feelings.
- Monitor evaluator: this member is a good judge who will see all options and points of view. Weaknesses: may lack drive and be overly critical.
- Teamworker: this is a cooperative and perceptive member of the group who will strive to calm troubled waters. Weaknesses: easily influenced by others and may be indecisive in a crisis.
- Implementer: this member is good at turning ideas into practical actions, disciplined, efficient, reliable and conservative. Weaknesses: may be somewhat inflexible and slow to take up new ideas.
- Completer: a painstaking, conscientious and anxious member of the group who looks for errors and omissions but tries to keep tasks on schedule. Weaknesses: can be a nit-picker who may worry unduly.
- Specialist: this member provides expert knowledge and skills. Weaknesses: tends to dwell on technicalities and overlooks the 'big picture' (for more detail see Belbin, 1993).

## Example

In an annual review meeting in a special school you may act as the 'specialist' in relation to the needs of a child with a specific language disorder where the rest of the team will look towards your specific expert knowledge. However, during the discussion of a child where you have only minimal involvement you may act as the 'completer', keeping the group on task with a more objective view of the situation.

## Leadership style

Leadership does not necessarily reside in a particular person or position, but may emerge in relation to the demands of the situation. This role may shift from one group member to another depending on the particular task being undertaken. For example in a Child Protection Team the Head of Social Services may be the leader in the context of a complex case conference. At other times the child's key worker (who could be any member of the team) may take a leadership role in the coordination of information and the day-to-day decisions affecting the particular child and his or her family.

In some teams there may be an appointed leader, who is given the authority and responsibility to ensure that certain tasks are completed. This authority may be given by the group itself, in terms of nominating a leader from within their ranks. More often they will have been appointed to this position by the organization responsible for the team (health trust, education department, etc.). There has been a considerable amount written about leadership styles, but it is now widely recognized that there is no one style that will be appropriate for all groups and tasks. Three commonly described styles of leadership, summarized in Table 5.2, are:

- *Authoritarian or directive:* this style of leader attempts to influence the rest of the group by using their positional power, often by directing them in what to do and how to do it. This approach can be extremely effective in an emergency, where there is little time to reach group consensus. However, this style of leadership can restrict the group's creativity and contribution to decision making and can lead to lack of commitment to the group process. You can probably remember situations where you have wished that someone would take the lead to move the meeting and decision making forward, but you may have lacked the confidence or have felt it inappropriate to take this lead yourself.
- *Democratic or participative:* this type of leader will seek and use the input of the group and will encourage them to take an active part in establishing policies and procedures within the team. Wherever possible, decisions are made on the basis of negotiation and consensus. This style of leadership can be very effective in obtaining and maintaining group commitment to the tasks in hand. This is often the style of leadership preferred by a team that works together frequently and has clear tasks that need to be completed. Group members are likely to feel that their ideas and contributions are valued and respected and are therefore more likely to participate actively within the group.
- *Laissez faire or non-directive:* this style is characterized by a deliberate effort not to interfere or intervene in the activities of the team. This approach can encourage the team members to be self-directed and flexible in their contribution to the process. This can be very effective for well-established teams who are highly skilled and self-motivated, but is often problematic for less experienced staff. The lack of defined leadership may lead to a lack of focus on the task in hand, so that group members may feel that valuable time is being wasted.

It is useful to consider what leadership qualities you view as important, and for the group as a whole to recognize the contribution made by different types of leaders.

**Table 5.2:** Styles of leadership

| Authoritarian | Democratic | Laissez faire |
|---|---|---|
| Directive | Participative | Non-directive |
| - good in emergency | - ensures all views are heard | - allows for individuality |
| - restricts creativity | - leads to agree solution | - hard for less established members |
| - may lead to lack of commitment | - difficult if very diverse opinions | - may be time consuming |

In many teams you may not be in a position of leadership, but your positive contribution to the team may be just as important. Therefore, it is also useful to consider the issue of 'followship'. Some important characteristics of a good follower include:

- ability to think for yourself
- knowledge of your own strengths and weaknesses
- clear understanding of the task and purpose of the group
- ability to express your own view clearly and objectively
- respect for the contribution and expertise of other members of the group
- being prepared to negotiate and compromise on some occasions.

### Decision-making strategies

The way a team comes to make decisions is often closely linked to the leadership style in operation. However, how the decision is reached can affect both the quality of the decision and individual members' commitment to it. Decisions may be reached in the following ways:

- *Individual decision,* where one individual may make the decision for the group. This may be made by the leader in their position of authority or may be because a certain team member has the relevant knowledge and expertise in that area. The leader's or team member's position and standing within the group may influence how well the group comply with or support the decision.
- *Minority decision* where, similar to individual decision making, a minority of the group members may make a decision on the basis of their expert position or knowledge. If this expertise is recognized and valued by the group, the decision is likely to be supported. However, if group members feel coerced into 'going along' with the decision, commitment to it is likely to be weakened. On some occasions, minority decisions may be pushed through because the majority may

be unaware that they are in fact in the majority. Hence the importance of a climate where all group members feel free to express their own views.

- *Majority vote.* This type of decision making is common when time is limited or when there are clear differences of opinion. Although this is likely to enlist majority support for the decision, the outvoted minority may feel less than committed to the decision or even strive to make it ineffective.
- *Consensus decision* making may be extremely time consuming, as all views will need to be fully aired and all perspectives and options discussed. However, the final decision is likely to have the commitment of most members of the team. It may not mean that all members agree fully with all aspects of the decision, but hopefully they will understand how it was reached, and accept enough to comply.

The type of decision making will be influenced by:

- leadership style
- the importance of the decision
- the expertise of the group
- the time allowed
- the climate and cohesion of the team.

### Purpose and tasks

Groups come together for a great variety of reasons. The purpose of the team is likely to influence the composition and working practice of the group members. The team may be established on a fairly permanent basis and the members may spend all or most of their work time as a member of the team. This may apply to a Child Development Team, Rehabilitation Centre team or staff working together in a special school. In other situations this team may be established on a temporary basis for the life of a particular project, such as developing a training package. At other times individuals may only be involved with the team for limited periods of their work, for example as part of a Feeding Assessment Team. Many speech and language clinicians may in fact work in a range of different teams during their working week. This may necessitate the ability to switch style and role very quickly and requires considerable flexibility, adaptability and assertiveness.

Much of the time and energy of the team is likely to be focused on the specific tasks allocated to them, that is the *task-oriented behaviours*, but it is also important to recognize that other issues may emerge during group meetings. Time may need to be focused on *maintenance behaviours* to build and sustain relationships among group members. These may be important in the reduction of tension and resolution of conflict, and to ensure the effective and coordinated contribution of group members. This has led to the development of 'team-building' exercises that may not be related to the tasks of the group, but which serve to establish and maintain good working relationships. Also within the team, members will have their own individual needs to be satisfied, such as the desire for recognition and success. These may lead to *self-oriented behaviours* that may cause unexpected stresses and a range of 'hidden agendas' that may impede the completion of the task. Again it may be important to address these issues outside of the focus on specific work tasks (see Table 5.3).

**Table 5.3:** Functions within the group

---

**Task-oriented functions**
*Initiating:* new ideas or ways of looking at the situation
*Information seeking:* asking appropriate questions
*Information giving:* clear statement of facts and opinions
*Opinion seeking:* openness to the views of others
*Opinion giving:* prepared to express our personal views
*Clarifying:* restating or questioning
*Elaborating:* expanding on points made by other members of the group
*Coordinating:* demonstrating relationship between different ideas and information
*Orienting:* checking on direction of discussion and keeping on task
*Testing:* checking that you clearly understand what has been said
*Summarizing:* drawing information together in a clear manner

**Maintenance functions**
*Encouraging:* being warm and friendly to other members of the group
*Mediating:* conciliating differences in opinion
*Gatekeeping:* helping others to make a contribution
*Standard-setting:* how groups, will operate, rules, choice of tasks, etc.
*Following:* serving as an audience for other group members
*Relieving tension:* diverting attention, smoothing over disagreements

**Self-oriented functions**
*Expressing own perspective*
*Defending professional or personal perspective*
*Maintaining own position*
*Gaining reinforcement and support*
*Preserving own role*

---

Adapted from Jaques (1991).

## Conflict

> A conflict exists when individuals, acting in their own best interests, participate in activities that generate tension. The tension results from significant disagreements or incompatible interests and activities (Wywialowski, 1993).

Generally conflict is viewed as negative, but *constructive conflict* that compels group members to examine their position can stimulate change and should therefore be encouraged. In contrast, *destructive conflict* will create stresses that will influence the quality of the work of the team.

Interpersonal and inter-group conflicts frequently originate from differences in personal or professional beliefs, values and working practices. Conflict can only be constructive if team members have a clear view of their common aims and understand the role and contribution of individual team members. Negative conflict that impedes the decision-making process needs to be addressed rather than ignored. Honest and open communication between team members needs to be fostered so that this type of conflict can be avoided. Johnson and Johnson (1991) suggest seven steps that may be useful to consider when trying to resolve conflict:

1. *Confront the opposition*: this allows you to express your own view of the problem and allows the opposition to do the same.
2. *Jointly define the conflict*: view it as a problem to be solved, rather than a situation of competition which someone must win. Try to define the problem as precisely and in as much detail as you can; this should then make it easier to manage.
3. *Communicate positions and feelings*: work together to understand each other's positions more clearly, and be open to change.
4. *Communicate cooperative intentions*: communicate and be sincere in your attempts to cooperate. Try not to be defensive, try to establish a shared goal and recognize that opposing views can be the basis for healthy exchange of ideas.
5. *Take the opponent's perspective*: this will give you greater understanding of why each person maintains their position, which may help in the process of reaching a satisfactory solution.
6. *Coordinate motivation to negotiate in good faith*: the benefits of negotiating a solution may outweigh the personal costs of conflict. To move towards a resolution hidden agendas must be exposed and honest negotiation must take place.
7. *Reach an agreement*: conflict is resolved when agreement satisfactory to all parties has been reached. This will probably involve compromise on all sides.

### The multidisciplinary team

Working in a range of team settings means that the speech and language clinician may need to take on a number of different roles and responsibilities. This may call for an understanding of the contributions and different perspectives of a wide variety of other people. This is not always easy, especially as at present unidisciplinary training may foster a 'professional culture' that encourages a competitive rather than a collaborative atmosphere. Frequently professionals may be unaware of their own particular professional background, which influences their working practice, and may have little awareness and understanding of the norms and practices of other professionals with whom they interact. As well as these professional influences there may also be organizational and agency differences that may further affect these relationships. For example a Child Protection Team may have representatives from social, education and health services, as well as the police and voluntary agencies, all with different organizational and managerial structures, and procedures. (This will be discussed in more detail later in the chapter.)

Collaborative practice is enhanced if professionals take time to consider their own professional perspective and gain an understanding of the personal, professional, organizational and agency influences affecting their colleagues. Huntington (1981) suggests a useful framework for compiling a 'Professional Profile' that might form a basis for discussion and comparison with others.

It may be helpful to consider the following questions yourself and then compare them with the responses gained from other professionals with whom you work:

- What is the overall 'mission statement' of your service?
- What are your key professional aims, for example is it to cure, teach, adapt, etc.?
- What is the core knowledge on which your profession is based?
- Do you use specific vocabulary that may be misunderstood by others?
- How do you view your relationship with your client? For example:
  - patient/doctor
  - pupil/teacher
  - client/consultant
  - facilitator.
- How do you usually relate to other professional groups?
  - receiving referrals
  - referring clients on
  - as a manager
  - collaboratively.

As mentioned in Chapter 1, research into the identification of the skills, knowledge and attitudes of the speech and language clinician has been carried out by van der Gaag and Davies (1992 a, b). This has been taken up by the Royal College of Speech and Language Therapists (RCSLT) in an attempt to define the core competencies of the profession. Similar projects are being undertaken by some other professional groups in the UK, such as physiotherapy and occupational therapy groups which will contribute to a greater understanding between professionals.

## The interdisciplinary and transdisciplinary team

If you are able to be a part of a team for extended periods of time you may be able to move towards true 'interdisciplinary' work, where there is joint planning and implementation of intervention. For example this may occur in a Child Development Centre where the various

pro-fessionals may run joint assessment or therapy sessions with each
professional's objectives being integrated to form a holistic programme of
management (see Figure 5.1).

---

**Example: Child with cerebral palsy**

The physiotherapist, speech and language clinician, and occupational therapist may coordinate their management plans so that all individuals working
with the child both inside and outside the centre are aware of the following:

* which postures and movements to encourage, and why
* which undesirable motor behaviours to discourage, and why
* which positions make it easier for the child to cooperate, move and
  communicate
* how to communicate with the child, and levels of communicative ability
* how to develop language and expression
* what sensory and perceptual difficulties are present, how material should be
  presented and what sensory and perceptual experiences to encourage
* what equipment is necessary to aid activities and how this should be used
* how to carry or move the child if necessary
* what toys, activities, etc. can be used to motivate the child and how these can
  be adapted to the child's problem.

---

Figure 5.1: Joint programme for a child with cerebral palsy.

Transdisciplinary working may emerge as professionals work alongside
each other and there is a transference of some skills between the professionals involved. This may occur in a Portage team where one professional
will be appointed to work directly with the child and the family, but may
carry out a range of types of therapy under the supervision of other professionals within the team. It will be important for such a team to have developed mutual trust and respect for each other's expertise. All group
members must be clear about the limitations of their skills and where
professional boundaries lie.

## Portage

A home-based teaching service for pre-school children with special needs.
Portage home visitors usually visit weekly and work with parents to plan activities so that their child learns new skills in small steps.

Wilson and Laidler (1990) describe a successful transdisciplinary
rehabilitation team. They highlight two significant factors that are central
to the team's success:

•  Respect for individuals' core expertise, knowledge and experience.
   This is seen to be specific to the professional and not shared with other
   disciplines.

**Table 5.4:** Skill blending

Example: for the child with cerebral palsy considered earlier

| Professions involved | Physiotherapy | Occupational therapy | Speech and language therapy |
|---|---|---|---|
| Core skills | Assessment of physical status Positioning and movement | Assessment of daily living skills Wheelchair assessment Switch access | Assessment for and introduction to AAC Considering communication options |
| Skill blending | Positioning for activities Lifting and carrying | Positioning of equipment Developing independence | Sign language Encouraging communication Turn-taking skills |

- The process of skill blending; through sharing of information and techniques particular to the individual client, certain skills are transmitted to other members of the team (see Table 5.4).

### Inter-agency initiatives

Many of the considerations discussed in previous sections will apply to the context of inter-agency collaboration. However, relationships and differences of 'cultural' background may be even more complex. Often these initiatives will be set up and formalized at a managerial level, but are likely to influence the work of everyone involved with the particular client group.

Hudson (1987) suggests that there are certain prerequisites to effective inter-agency collaborative activity:

1. *Inter-organizational homogeneity*: this is the degree to which all members share a functional and structural similarity. Major differences at this level can lead to tension and conflict.
2. *Domain consensus*: this arises from the need for clear agreement on the expectations of what the team can and cannot do. This requires:
   (a) agreement on specific goals
   (b) compatibility of organizational goals, philosophies and orientation
   (c) agreement of the hierarchy within the venture.
3. *Network awareness*: this requires positive evaluation and respect for the work of other agencies and organisations.
4. *Organizational exchange*: it is important that interactions are based on reciprocal reinforcement. Involvement in the collaboration must have positive benefits for all the agencies involved, although this does not have to be on an equal basis. No group should be powerless in relation to others.

5. *Alternative resource sources*: the availability of 'outside' sources of finance or human resources may weaken the incentive for agencies to become involved or committed to working with others.

In many situations there may be a 'lead' agency that will take overall responsibility for the venture. However, working in such a way as to satisfy the needs of more than one agency can be very demanding. A clear framework of collaboration may need to be formalized in order that the group can move forward in an effective manner.

All the considerations described above may seem to make the idea of team or multidisciplinary working rather complex and threatening, but with thought and planning it can lead to very exciting and challenging experiences. However, you do need to make sure that you are clear about your own role and expectations before you begin. You need to develop good interpersonal skills so that you can put your own views across in a clear and assertive manner. Teamwork will inevitably require compromise, but when you get it right it can lead to enhanced and coordinated client care as well as great personal satisfaction.

In most of this discussion the client may have been seen as peripheral to the team, but it is obvious that in relation to his or her own particular situation he or she is the 'key player'who should, whenever possible, be the prime decision maker. It is important to explore ways in which the client's voice can be clearly heard. As discussed in Chapter 1, the role of the 'patient' has been changing over the past 20 or 30 years. They are now more frequently considered as a customer or consumer of services, rather than in the traditional 'medical model' of care where they have been viewed as passive recipients of services. If we are truly to work in partnership with our clients we must enable them to voice their opinions and be aware of the professional power we hold:

> ...the professional's world view no longer takes precedence over the client's. Nor does the professional have the right to set the terms of the relationship, to prescribe behaviour and to expect compliance. The relationship is now a negotiated one; and the role of the professional is to develop an understanding of his/her client's perceived needs, and to share his/her expert knowledge and skills, in so far as they serve these needs (Williams, 1993: 14).

## The speech and language team

The speech and language department may consist of the following staff groups:

* speech and language clinicians
* speech and language assistants
* bilingual co-workers
* administrative staff.

Although each group will have different job priorities and backgrounds, the various members will hopefully work together often enough to develop a shared culture.

### The speech and language clinician

The opportunity to work with other speech and language clinicians is often a stimulating and rewarding experience. Here the same educational and professional backgrounds are shared, resulting in easy understanding of each other's working methods and terminology. As well as the obvious 'two heads are better than one' advantage, other gains might include:

- one clinician being able to focus on observing and recording data while the other conducts the activity with the client
- use of a colleague as a role model of desired behaviour
- learning from the expertise of a more experienced clinician
- viewing the client from two different perspectives or specialisms
- sharing the workload of administration, report writing, etc.
- providing and receiving feedback on performance, language levels, etc.
- observing and experimenting with different approaches
- ability to focus attention on the needs of both the client and their relative/carer.

As well as working together directly, contact with others in the same profession is extremely important in terms of emotional and professional support. Rose describes how clinical isolation resulted in her becoming extremely disillusioned with the job, such that she contemplated leaving the profession altogether (Hawkins and Shohet, 1992). It is feared that the continuing changes in the health service, the loss of professional managed services and changing employment conditions may lead to further fragmentation of departments resulting in even greater isolation of professionals. The RCSLT acknowledges that all newly qualified speech and language clinicians should have access to a mentoring system. Regular contact with a more experienced colleague should be timetabled into their programme. More formal supervision is also being offered to all levels of staff in some departments. This practice, well established in the social work profession, has only recently been recognized as important by other professional groups (for further discussion see Chapter 8).

However, there are also a number of other avenues that can be used to maintain contact and gain support from other members of the profession:

- membership of the professional body giving access to regular newsletters, journals, etc.
- membership of local networks of clinicians
- Special Interest Groups, where clinicians working within the same area of specialty or with a developing interest in that area come together to share ideas and concerns

- attendance at staff meetings
- establishing local journals club, where colleagues get together to discuss recent research
- attendance on courses and at conferences
- audit groups and peer review
- union membership
- joint projects with colleagues.

The role you play as a speech and language clinician will vary considerably within the contexts in which you are working. Roulstone (1988), a speech and language therapist working in a special school for children with severe learning difficulties, suggests that clinicians operate in at least three distinct roles:

1. *Coordinator* of all aspects of communication. This may involve coordinating language groups, working with assistants and other personnel.
2. *Skills transmitter*. This may be done on a one-to-one basis in the classroom, or through more formalized training sessions, such as teaching sign language to all staff in the school/centre.
3. *Participant*. It is important that the clinician is seen as an integral part of the work environment. It may be important to participate in a wide range of curricular and extracurricular activities. This will enable them to model and encourage appropriate communication strategies and establish credibility within the team.

These roles may be seen to be appropriate to any setting, where there will be a need to balance the various aspects to provide an effective and valued service.

With continuing pressure on resources, the speech and language clinician is increasingly required to act in the role of advisor or consultant, with less direct contact with the clients themselves. Egan (1978) gives a useful definition of consultancy:

The CONSULTANT influences the TARGET via the efforts of a MEDIATOR.

In this context the mediator may be the teacher, nurse, assistant, parent or volunteer. The speech and language clinician will remain responsible for the assessment and identification of goals and objectives, but much of the intervention may be carried out by others in the client's environment. This may necessitate the writing of detailed and clear programmes that can be left for others to carry out. Success will rely heavily on the quality of the relationships established with key staff. Regular contact to review and monitor programmes and provide training and support for staff will be vital.

## Speech and language assistants

Speech and language assistants have been employed in Great Britain for many years. However, this has mostly been on an individual basis to work with clearly defined client groups, for example working with stroke groups, in special schools, etc. Speech and language assistants are not required to hold any formal qualification prior to employment but will work under the direction of a qualified clinician. In the UK, National Occupational Standards have now been defined (Care Sector Consortium, 1996) and these have formed the basis of the National and Scottish Vocational qualifications (S/NVQ) Care Awards at Level 3. This is equivalent to a university entrance level qualification The RCSLT has established programmes and assessment criteria for this award so that assistants can work towards a recognized qualification.

A survey carried out by the UK Association of Speech Therapy Managers in 1989 established that 34 per cent of health districts employed assistants, although numbers ranged from one to six per district. Assistants appeared to be most commonly working with children and also with adults with learning disabilities. Although the number of assistants at this time was quite small, there is evidence of a gradual increase in these numbers that may be further accelerated as NVQ standards become more established.

The speech and language assistant can be a vital member of the team. Although they may have had little or no formal training, they may bring a wealth of relevant experience to the role. However, it is important to be clear about what you can expect of them (Table 5.5), and also your management and training responsibility towards them. You must remember that you remain responsible for client care even when you have delegated some of the more routine aspects of management to the assistant.

Make sure that you are always clear about what you expect them to do, and that there are well-established channels of communication. You may leave detailed instructions or programmes to be carried out by the assistant, but it will also be important for them to work alongside you on some occasions. They will also need to understand the overall aims of the programmes of intervention you are following. They will need feedback on their own performance and how they have influenced the behaviour of the clients they are working with.

**Table 5.5**: Role of assistants

| What assistants do | What assistants don't do |
| --- | --- |
| Carry out routine therapy tasks | In-depth assessment |
| Help with routine administration tasks, e.g. photocopying, etc. | Answer questions put by carers or other professionals |
| Prepare therapy materials | Work unsupervised |
| Keep records about therapy undertaken | Write reports |

The guidelines in Table 5.6 may help the speech and language clinician to ensure that the assistants (or others working with the client) are confident about what they are doing.

**Table 5.6:** Guidelines for teaching therapy procedures to others

1. Specify desired behaviour and outcome clearly, and explain *why* it is important.
2. Outline procedure and the rationale for its design.
3. Explain sequence of steps involved.
4. Demonstrate the sequence with the client involved.
5. Ask assistant to review/describe the demonstration, reinforce and clarify the procedure.
6. Provide the opportunity for the assistant to demonstrate procedure on you or another member of staff if appropriate.
7. Observe assistant carrying out procedure with client, provide feedback and correct *only* critical aspects of the procedure.
8. Review, discuss and revise as necessary, providing written notes to act as prompt. Discuss and agree how progress is going to be monitored and recorded.
9. Encourage assistant to initiate questions and make contact as necessary.
10. Arrange date and time for review and follow-up.

## Bilingual co-workers

Bilingual services for clients with speech and language disorders are being established, particularly in areas with large populations of people from black and ethnic minority groups.

The bilingual co-worker will usually be recruited from the local community and is employed and trained by the speech and language department. As well as having in-depth knowledge of the community language(s), they may also be able to provide a wealth of knowledge about cultural issues and the local community.

The RCSLT guidelines (RCSLT, 1996) suggest the co-worker may fulfil the following roles:

- gathering case history information from the client or carer in their home language
- assessing and observing the client in their mother tongue
- contributing to the differential diagnosis between a primary language disorder and difficulties arising from English as a second language
- contributing to the management and therapy of clients whose first language is not English
- interpreting information between the client and the professional
- offering written information in the client's mother tongue as appropriate
- advising on culturally appropriate play and clinical materials.

Not all departments will employ such workers, and even those who are able to may not have resources to employ co-workers speaking all the languages used in the local community. If an appropriate co-worker is not available, then try:

- borrowing the services of a co-worker from a neighbouring trust
- using the facilities of other local interpreting services. These are often available through NHS trust or education/social departments
- seeking the advice of a specialist or advisor on bilingualism, or contact an appropriate Special Interest Group.

### Administrative staff

Secretarial and administrative staff will be central to the smooth running of a speech and language department. They are likely to be the first point of contact for the client and their family, through sending out appointments, taking phone inquiries and messages, and receiving clients at the clinic. It is important that such staff have some understanding of the communication problems these clients may experience, and have developed good interpersonal skills in order to make clients feel welcome and at ease.

Such staff may also be responsible for:

- typing letters and reports
- maintaining client records
- inputting statistical information on to the computer
- maintenance and recording of equipment and resources.

It is vital that they observe issues of client confidentiality and understand the sensitivity of the information they handle.

## Summary

The newly qualified clinician has many avenues for professional support and advice. Some of this will be through formalized networks, but much can also be gained through less formal means. Being open to the suggestions of others and listening to discussions that take place in the department will provide invaluable information. You should also realize the importance of the support and information you can bring to the department and be prepared to express your own views and discuss your own experiences.

# Chapter 6
# Working in Different
# Settings

As discussed in Chapter 5, the speech and language clinician will work in a range of different settings and interact and collaborate with staff from a variety of agencies. In the UK, speech and language clinicians are usually employed by the National Health Service, so some staff may work in a wide variety of health care settings. However, other members of the department may find that the majority of their contact is with non-health professionals.

## Working in health settings

The service may be organized as a separate department managed by a speech and language manager as part of a clinical directorate, or the manager may be a clinical coordinator responsible for a number of professional groups. In the latter case the manager may not be a speech and language clinician. In small departments there may be only one speech and language clinician within this team, and she may have little professional contact with others with the same background, as shown in Figure 6.1.

The most common health care settings are:

- hospitals
- child development centres
- rehabilitation centres
- community clinics/health centres.

### General hospitals

Work here may involve contact with both inpatients and outpatients. Inpatient care may include work on the ward as well as seeing clients who are brought to the department. It is essential that all other professionals involved with the client are aware of the input of the speech and language service and any relevant information that they have about the client. This exchange of information and liaison may take place through:

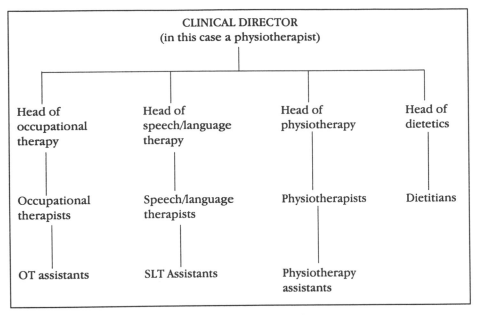

**Figure 6.1:** Example of the organization of a therapy department.

- informal discussion amongst staff
- attendance on ward rounds
- notes kept in the patient's medical file
- information kept in the nurses' Cardex/care plan system
- through liaison with the primary nurse involved with the client
- letters and reports sent to referring agents, etc.
- case conferences and ward meetings.

*The ward setting*

The hospital ward is invariably a busy place with many different professionals all needing to carry out important tasks in relation to the patient. It is important that we introduce ourselves to the person with day-to-day responsibility for the ward. This is usually the charge nurse or sister. We should then negotiate a suitable time and space to work with the patient. Many wards now have unrestricted visiting so we also need to be sensitive to the needs of family and friends.

Private space is often at a premium, so some consultations may need to take place at the bedside, with maybe only a curtain between the patient and the rest of the ward. This can be quite a distracting environment and there may be little privacy for confidential case history taking and personal discussion.

Some patients, particularly if they are required to spend more than a few days in hospital, may become somewhat 'institutionalized' by the process. Signs of this may include:

- passivity and over compliance
- inability to make decisions
- depression and lack of motivation.

This is likely to have consequences on their response to any intervention and may give a false impression of their attitudes to communication and recovery.

## The outpatients department

Here the clinician may have more control over the timing of appointments for both clients who are inpatients and will have to be transported from the ward by porter staff, and clients who are outpatients and may require ambulance or hospital transport. However, these clients may still be involved with a number of hospital personnel and there may be a need for careful scheduling so that they do not have to make unnecessary trips to the hospital.
There are several points to consider:

- Can a joint appointment with other therapy staff be made? For example coordinated with physiotherapy or occupational therapy?
- Can the client cope with this level of input or is this too fatiguing?
- Is the order of appointments important? For example, relaxation carried out by the physiotherapist may have positive effects on the subsequent speech and language programme.
- Is this the most effective setting for therapy? Or would the client be more responsive if he or she was seen at home?

Within the outpatient department, the speech and language clinician is likely to have access to a greater variety of materials and a quieter environment for assessment and confidential discussion than on the ward. However, more effort may be needed to liaise and discuss clients with other staff and to keep ward notes up to date.

## Domiciliary visits

How much opportunity the speech and language therapist will have to undertake domiciliary visits will depend on:

- the policy of the department
- the geographical area
- the facilities available within the hospital
- the need for specialist equipment only available within the department
- the experience and level of supervision required by the therapist.

The home environment may hold advantages for the client and provides the opportunity for the therapist to:

- see clients when they are relaxed and at the best time of day
- observe the clients' communication skills in a functional setting
- have close contact with relatives and carers
- plan intervention which is relevant to the clients' everyday needs and environment.

Clinicians need to be aware of the additional time and organization that may be needed to travel around the locality and the necessity of having the materials they need for assessment and intervention with them. They also need to be aware of the potential risk that may be involved with seeing clients away from a centre where there are other staff on hand. Before undertaking a domiciliary visit clinicians should:

- check the department policy in relation to domiciliary visits and discuss this with their manager
- carry and wear an identification badge
- consider the level of potential risk involved with a particular client or setting
- consider whether the planned procedure may pose a potential risk to the client, for example an assessment for dysphagia
- be aware of safety procedures relevant to home visits, for example dealing with challenging behaviour or medical emergencies
- make sure that someone at the base knows where they are visiting and, if necessary, arrange to contact the base on the completion of the visit
- where necessary, arrange to visit with another professional.

**Child development centre (CDC)**

These centres provide a central focus for the assessment, or assessment and treatment, of children with complex needs. These teams are usually coordinated by a consultant paediatrician, and will also employ a range of therapists and a clinical psychologist, and may include representatives from social services and education. The majority of children seen at these centres are likely to be below the age of 5 years, although some centres also cater for school-aged children.

*The multidisciplinary assessment*

Instead of having to visit several different professionals for individual appointments, the child and their family may be offered an extended appointment when all the relevant professionals may be available. Once the assessment has been completed there will be a multiprofessional conference, usually including the parents, at which a coordinated plan of care and therapy will be decided. This therapy may take place within the CDC, again limiting the number of appointments that the family has to keep. In other centres the recommendations of the team will be passed on to local clinicians so that intervention takes place in the child's locality, but with the supervision and support of the specialist team. Many centres may also run multidisciplinary groups where, for example, speech and language therapy, physiotherapy and other disciplines provide input to a group of children attending the same session.

This setting can also provide the child's parents with the opportunity to meet and talk with other families who may be experiencing similar problems, and may be a useful source of general advice and information for the community clinician.

### Rehabilitation centres

These centres are designed to provide intensive therapeutic rehabilitation, and clients may either be residential or attend on a daily basis. The main aims of the service are to help clients to reach their full potential and to maximize long-term functioning. Referral to the centre is usually via medical personnel and the centre is likely to be managed by a consultant. As well as in-depth assessment of communication and swallowing disorders, the speech and language clinician may be involved with other disciplines in the assessment of related skills. For example:

- SLT and physiotherapy: posture, breathing and voice production
- SLT and occupational therapy: writing and accessing of augmentative and alternative communication (AAC) devices
- SLT and psychologist: cognition, reasoning, memory skills.

Following the multidisciplinary assessment, what is known as a joint report and care plan will be drawn up by the team in consultation with the client and his or her carers. This plan may then be instituted within the rehabilitation centre, where intensive therapy input can be arranged, or less intensive therapy may be arranged on an outpatient or domiciliary basis.

### Community clinics/health centres

The health centre is the base for the primary health care team, and is usually the client's first and main access to medical services.

> Primary care is the provision of integrated, accessible health care services by clinicians who are accountable for addressing a large majority of personal health care needs, developing a sustained partnership with patients, and practising in the context of family and community (Institute of Medicine, 1996).

This team is usually controlled and coordinated by the GP, who will be the gatekeeper to a range of other medical services, including referral to specialist medical personnel. Increasingly in Great Britain, GPs have become fundholders, responsible for the control and allocation of a budget with which they can purchase health care directly from health care providers, rather than having it purchased on their behalf by their district health authority. Their budget is allocated from central government on a per capita basis. Speech and language services have striven to preserve an open referral system, so that potential clients have direct access to services. However, with the growth in the number of fundholding practices, this has become increasingly difficult to maintain. It is essential that the GP is kept informed of the speech and language clinician's involvement with their clients, and this should be done through copies of letters to acknowledge referral, reports written after assessment, interim and discharge reports. The 1997 White Paper *The New NHS* recommends the phasing out of GP fundholding, but this will be replaced by teams of GPs and nurses in Primary Care Groups who will shape services for their clients.

Although in theory any client may access speech and language services through their local health centre, in practice the majority of referrals will comprise pre-school children. In some areas children may continue to be seen at their local clinic after they have started school, whereas in other areas they are likely to have their management transferred to a clinician who visits and works in their school. Some clinicians may be happy to assess and work with a wider client group, for example adults with learning disabilities and adults discharged from hospital, but less experienced staff may wish to pass these referrals on to the relevant specialists.

*Child surveillance*

Historically, in the UK the monitoring of the development of the pre-school child has been undertaken by the health visitor, and so many early referrals to speech and language services have come from this source. The *Health for All Children* document (Hall, 1989) outlined contractual arrangements for regular child surveillance to be undertaken by GPs. This includes special payment for all surveillance activity undertaken in an attempt to motivate practices to take a more organized and proactive approach to child health. It is suggested that children have general checks at:

- 7–10 days
- 6 weeks
- 7–9 months, to include screening of hearing and vision
- 18–24 months, to include speech and understanding
- 36–42 months, to include a developmental assessment.

Surveillance should also include screening as a result of parental concern and follow-up of children who fail to thrive. As this practice becomes more established it may well impact on how and when children are referred to a speech and language service.

## Other personnel working in hospitals, clinics and health centres

### The clinical director

This may be a doctor, nurse or member of the paramedical professions who heads up the clinical directorate and who will have both clinical and managerial responsibilities. They may have responsibility for a number of different professionals within the directorate and will represent their views to the Chief Executive.

### Medical staff

### Consultant

This is the most senior doctor working within the hospital, who will be ultimately responsible for the patient's medical care. He or she will be a specialist in their particular area of medicine, for example orthopaedics, oncology or geriatric medicine. He or she may be the source of referral of in- or outpatients and will need to be kept fully informed of your involvement. He or she will be supported by junior doctors, such as senior registrars and house officers, who are training to become consultants or GPs.

### The general practitioner

The GP will be the leader of the primary health care team and will be responsible for all decisions made about the patients on their list. He or she is an important source of information and referral. It is important that he or she is kept fully informed of your involvement with their patients.

### Nursing staff

### Charge nurse/sister

This is the person responsible for the day-to-day care of the patients on his or her ward. He or she is responsible for the allocation of nursing duties and the overall organization of ward staff.

### Primary nurse

In many hospitals the patient will be assigned to a primary nurse who takes responsibility for a named group of patients. He or she will be responsible for coordinating the patient's care and liaising with relatives and other professionals as necessary.

### The health visitor

This is a fully qualified nurse who has undergone additional training. She or he may work particularly with young families and, along with the GP, is responsible for the routine surveillance of children up to the age of 5 years. The health visitor's regular contact with families means that she or he is frequently the primary referring agency for pre-school children to the speech and language service, and will usually be able to provide detailed background information on the child and the family.

## The practice nurse

As well as carrying out many routine nursing activities within the centre, the practice nurse may run special clinics for particular groups of patients suffering from conditions such as diabetes and asthma. The practice nurse can be an extremely useful source of information about particular patients, and needs to be kept informed of our involvement.

## The district nurse

The district nurse will provide nursing care and support to people in their homes, and may be a useful source of information. She or he may be particularly involved with a patient immediately after discharge from hospital and will be aware of social as well as medical aspects of the patient's condition.

## The community nurse

The community nurse will usually have specific training in relation to learning disability. She or he will be a primary point of contact and support for the client with learning disability and their family, and will also provide information on medical needs, financial benefits and local resources, and, where appropriate, will arrange for referral to other relevant profes-sionals. There may also be designated nurses who are specialists in dealing with particular client groups, such as those presenting with challenging behaviour.

## Other staff

### Physiotherapists

They use special skills and techniques to help people who are physically disabled by injury or illness to achieve as normal and active a life as is possible. They may work in hospitals, health centres, clinics, schools or people's homes, and they provide a service to all ages.

### Occupational therapists

Their aim is to help people to achieve and maintain the maximum degree of independence possible in all aspects of their daily lives. This may involve teaching different ways of doing everyday tasks, supplying special equipment or recommending adaptation to housing, etc. They work with all age ranges and may be employed within the health service or by the social services department.

### Dietitians

They may work within the hospital or be based in the community. They aim to promote health and prevent disease by giving dietary and nutritional advice to patients and staff. They are likely to be involved in the management of children and adults with swallowing difficulties and can advise on suitable textures and food supplements.

### Clinical psychologists

They are trained in the assessment and treatment of psychological problems. They provide a service for people of all ages with a wide range of health problems, in particular those with learning disabilities, elderly people and children and adults with mental health problems. Their aim is to help people to develop more effective ways of coping with problems and illness, and in the management of problem behaviour.

### The practice manager

They are likely to be responsible for the day-to-day running of the health centre, and will organize such things as room availability, resources, security, etc. If you are working within the clinic it is important to negotiate access and keep the manager informed of your activities.

### Administrative staff

They will be a vital source of information and may be responsible for some of your administration tasks, such as typing reports, sending out appointments, etc. In other situations all administration will go through a central speech and language office. Wherever you are based, it is important that a member of staff is aware of your activities at all times. This is for your own personal safety. For example, if you undertake a home visit you should let someone know where you are going and at what time you should be expected back. The receptionist will also be the first line of contact for your clients and should therefore have the information needed to keep the clients informed.

## Working in education settings

In some countries speech and language clinicians may be employed directly by the education department or school. However, in the UK, most speech and language services in schools are provided by the local NHS trust, although increasingly trusts and local education authorities are entering into joint funding arrangements, whereby the NHS trust will retain overall responsibility for a service that is partly financed by the education department. However, it is recognized that there is often a significant shortfall between the amount of therapy provided and what the local education authority (LEA) would like (Council of Local Education Authorities, 1994). This has resulted in services and clinicians having to develop a range of innovative working practices and a need for good cooperation and support from school staff. Jowett and Evans (1996) have published an extremely interesting and useful account of their research into collaborative practice between speech and language therapists and teachers. They also suggest a useful framework for collaborative practice.

There has been considerable change to the organization of the education system in the UK, as a result of a range of legislation during the late 1980s and the 1990s.

1. 1988: The Education Reform Act. This far-reaching legislation involved:
   - the implementation of the National Curriculum, and national assessment arrangements
   - the introduction of local management of schools (LMS), which gives schools greater budgetary and decision-making control
   - an increase in the powers and responsibilities of school governors
   - the introduction of open enrolment, allowing parents greater choice over school placement.
2. 1992: The Office For Standards in Education (OFSTED) was set up to inspect, report and improve the standards of achievement and quality in schools by a 4-year cycle of school inspection. Also school league tables were introduced and published allowing parents to compare school attainment and examination results.
3. 1993: The Funding Agency for Schools in England, and the Schools Funding Council for Wales, were established, to take over responsibility for planning school places within their areas.
4. 1994: There was a streamlining of the National Curriculum and assessment arrangements to make it more manageable. The core subjects are now English, maths and science.
5. 1996: Legislation was introduced to raise the standards in schools by encouraging schools to take greater responsibility for achieving high standards, by setting targets and accounting for performance. This included an extension of LMS so that schools control 95 per cent of the budget, although the financing of children with Statements of Educational Need still remains with the LEA.
6. 1997: A consultative paper was published that aimed to increase inclusion of children with special educational needs. It also sought to provide speech and language therapy more effectively for the children

who needed it and encouraged the more effective and widespread use of information and communication technology to support their education.

In relation to children with special needs, the 1981 Education Act has provided the foundation for services for children with special needs in the UK. This defined special educational needs as:

> ...a child has special educational needs if he has a learning difficulty which calls for special educational provision to be made for him ... and a child has a 'learning difficulty' if ... he has a significantly greater difficulty in learning than the majority of children of his age. (DES, 1981)

The Warnock Report (1978), the predecessor to the 1981 Act, suggested that between 18 and 20 per cent of children would have some sort of special educational need at some stage of their school career. At this time special schools were catering for approximately 2 per cent of the school population. Other aspects of the Act promoted an integrated education service for these children, and introduced the concept of the 'Statement of Educational Need'. This is a legal document drawn up by the LEA in consultation with parents and the professionals involved with the child. It outlines the child's special educational needs and the resources necessary to meet these needs. As a result of this legislation and the commitment to a policy of integration, some special schools closed and the majority of others underwent a significant change in their character and organization. However, the Warnock committee envisaged that there would always be a small core of children who would require segregated school provision.

During the 1980s and early 1990s there was a steady rise in the number of children being given the protection of a Statement (Table 6.1). This had obvious resource implications. Although the principles introduced by the 1981 Act have been maintained, the process has been revised by the introduction of the Code of Practice on the Identification and Assessment of Special Educational Needs (Department of Education and Science, 1993). This clearly outlines the assessment and statementing procedure, and identifies the school's and LEA responsibilities in relation to this process. It also aims to limit the issuing of a Statement to those children who require resources beyond those usually available in the mainstream school. This aims to focus these additional resources on the 2 per cent of children who have severe and/or complex needs. The Code of Practice also introduced a new appeals and tribunal procedure for parents who are unhappy with the decisions made by the LEA.

## Children with speech and language difficulties in mainstream education

There are likely to be a number of children in mainstream schools who will require the attention of a speech and language clinician. They can be divided into two groups.

**Table 6.1:** Percentage of pupils with a Statement

|  | 1983/84 | 1993/94 | 1994/95 |
|---|---|---|---|
| % of all pupils with a Statement | 2.00 | 2.4 | 2.7 |

From 1997 Green Paper, *Education For Excellence*.

## *Statemented children*

These will usually be the children with the more severe and complex needs, who have undergone the full assessment process. Many of these children will have severe communication difficulties and may require the input of a speech and language clinician. There has been considerable debate over whether such provision should be included in the Statement under Part 6, Non-educational provision, or under Part 3, Educational provision. High Court judgement (R. v. Harrow London Borough Council) placed the responsibility for providing speech and language therapy in the hands of the local education authorities and thus made them legally responsible for ensuring its provision. It is important that the speech and language clinician working in schools is fully conversant with this legislation and Code of Practice, and that they consider the educational implications of the child's communication difficulties (see IPSEA p. 222).

## *Non-Statemented children*

Many children with communication difficulties will not fall into this 2 per cent, and the educational needs of these children will have to be met by the resources available within the school. Some speech and language services have a policy of providing help and support to all schoolchildren within the school setting. Others will provide support only to those children in possession of a Statement, with other children being catered for as clients at the local community clinic or health centre.

## Children with speech and language difficulties in special schools

The Warnock Report (1978) was keen to abolish categories of disability and replace them with an overarching definition of learning disability. However, there is still a wide range of categories of special schools both within local authorities and within the independent sector. There are schools catering for children with:

1. Sensory impairment:
   - visual impairment
   - hearing impairment.
2. Physical disabilities, including neurological and medical problems.

3. Emotional and behavioural difficulties.
4. Learning disabilities:
   - specific learning disabilities, e.g. developmental dyslexia
   - moderate learning disabilities
   - severe/profound learning disabilities.
5. Speech and language disabilities.

It should be remembered that children may have a range of difficulties and it may be difficult to decide which type of environment best meets all their needs.

When working in any school on a regular basis, it is important that everyone is clear about how this will be arranged. It is useful to meet with the headteacher and special needs coordinator to negotiate arrangements before the block of visits begins. For inexperienced staff it is useful to have a more senior speech and language clinician or manager present at this initial meeting. The areas that need to be discussed at this stage include:

- Who will you be working with?
    all children with speech and language problems
    only those with Statements.
- How will new referrals be handled?
- What do school staff expect of you? Is this realistic?
- What do you expect of school staff? Again, is this realistic?
- Where will you work?
- When will you be in school?
- Who will be your main point of contact and liaison?
    the special needs coordinator
    an assistant
    the head teacher.
- Will you have a fixed schedule of appointments?
- When will you be able to meet with school staff to discuss individual children?
- Who will be responsible for carryover work and implementing programmes?

It is useful to document these decisions and provide all interested partners with a copy, so that there can be no misunderstandings about these key issues. This does not mean that the arrangements cannot be changed, but this should be done through a process of consultation on both sides, rather than by decisions being made unilaterally.

### Speech and language intervention within the school

The main roles of the speech and language clinician within the school are likely to include:

- assessment
- direct intervention
- provision of programmes
- staff training
- contribution to school policies.

*Assessment*

The communication difficulties of many children will have been identified in the pre-school years. However, there are likely to be a number whose speech and language problems have not become apparent until they have been expected to meet the challenges of the classroom situation. This may be because they have been able to establish good interaction with familiar adults or their difficulties in intelligibility may only arise when they are in a situation where they have to communicate with less familiar people. For some children, language difficulties may be revealed when they are seen to struggle with some of the speaking and listening targets of the National Curriculum, or when they have difficulty with the development of early reading and writing skills. Another group often not identified until they reach school age are those children with pragmatic difficulties who may exhibit great difficulty establishing peer relationships.

For these reasons, the speech and language clinician working in mainstream schools can expect to receive a number of new referrals who will need assessment. It is important that parents have given clear consent prior to any involvement with the child. It is good practice to seek the parents' views and feelings about their child's difficulty by inviting them, wherever possible, to be a part of the assessment process.

There will also be a need for ongoing assessment and reassessment of children as they progress though the school system. The Code of Practice recommends the drawing up of an Individual Education Plan for any child experiencing difficulty in the classroom. This should include aims and objectives relating to speech and language development and will need to be reviewed and revised on a regular basis (see example in Figure 6.2).

Any child who is the subject of a school-based Individual Education Plan or Statement of Educational Need will have their progress reviewed and monitored on a regular basis. The speech and language clinician will be required to provide reports on the child's progress in communication and will be invited to participate in the annual review process.

*Direct intervention*

There are likely to be a small number of children whom the speech and language clinician may wish to work with directly on a regular basis. However, even if most of the intervention is being carried out by others, it will still be important to monitor progress directly in some way. There will always remain a need for the clinician to work directly with the client on some occasions:

| NAME: John B. | YEAR: 2 |
|---|---|

**Language and communication: (including English)**
1. Develop John's reading skills to a point where his reading age is within 2 years of his chronological age

2. Increase his understanding of instructions incorporating 4 or more information carrying words

**Academic development (including maths, science and foundation subjects)**
Count and give amounts of money up to £5

**Visuo-motor development**
Hit a tennis ball thrown from 3 metres, with a flat bat 6/10 times

**Social and emotional development**
1. Relay verbal messages to others within school
2. Play a board game with another child for at least 5 minutes without adult intervention

**Notes**
A programme will be provided by the speech and language therapist, and implemented three times a week by the SNA

**Medical factors**
John's epilepsy is being monitored. All staff should be advised of what to do in case of a fit

**Teacher's name:**                                                          **Date:**

**Signature:**

**Figure 6.2:** An Individual Education Plan (IEP).

- for further assessment
- for review and report writing
- at the request of other team members
- when the clinician is unsure about how to proceed with the client
- to demonstrate procedures and techniques to others
- when using specific equipment and techniques
- to maintain a relationship with the client
- to establish and maintain credibility within the team.

On some occasions the speech and language clinician may wish to withdraw children into a quiet one-to-one situation. Increasingly, however, visiting professionals are recognizing the importance of working within the child's natural environment, rather than working in an isolated one-to-one setting (the traditional broom cupboard). The benefits of working within the classroom include:

- assessing and identifying the child's strengths and weaknesses in the educational setting
- aims and objectives are more likely to be relevant to the child's everyday needs
- therapy is seen as part of the educational process and is made relevant to the classroom activities and environment
- other personnel can be more easily involved in the programme and the clinician can model appropriate strategies
- similarly the clinician is exposed to the strategies of other personnel (for example in relation to behaviour management)
- the clinician is also likely to be made aware of the pressures experienced within a busy classroom, so can tailor her demands accordingly
- language skills are more likely to generalize if they are integrated into the environment where natural cues occur.

Teachers are not always keen to welcome other professionals into the classroom. A survey by Gipps, Gross and Goldstein (1987) investigated teachers' attitudes to the range of support being provided for children with special needs in mainstream classrooms. They found that withdrawal by specially trained staff was viewed more favourably than assistance in the classroom or in-service training. It was felt that this was partly a reflection of previously established working practices, but also indicated a feeling of a lack of experience and expertise in dealing with these children. There was also a reluctance to accept responsibility for their needs. Although there has been a considerable investment in in-service training and changes in attitudes during the past few years, visiting professionals must be sensitive to the teacher's situation. They should be aware of the lack of in-depth training and experience in communication, the demands of a large and diverse class and the range of other responsibilities of the class teacher. Working practice should be clearly discussed and sensitively negotiated between all personnel involved. Finally it should not be forgotten that there may be advantages in withdrawing the child from the classroom on some occasions:

- It provides an opportunity for the child to spend time with an adult in what may be a more relaxed and less stressful environment.
- Some children may be very sensitive to failing in front of their peers, so may be reluctant to experiment with new skills within the classroom.
- A child with attention difficulties may need the opportunity to work in a quiet environment on some occasions.
- Assessment to compare 'optimum' ability with 'functional' ability may be useful.
- Some procedures (for example oral examinations) may need to be done in a private setting to preserve dignity.
- The therapist may be unsure of a procedure and may need to experiment in a less open environment.

- A procedure may require the use of specialist equipment unsuitable to the classroom environment.
- Certain therapy procedures may be highly distracting and not appropriate to the classroom setting.
- Likewise some class activities may not be conducive to focusing on the needs of one particular child.

### Provision of programmes to be carried out by school personnel

Increasingly, speech and language clinicians are working within a consultative model in schools, where they may have much less 'hands on' experience than was traditionally the case. This requires the development of a different range of skills, and success is dependent on good interpersonal relationships and the ability to negotiate with all involved. If the child has the protection of a Statement this may include the allocation of extra teaching or non-teaching assistance, and this may even be specified as time for speech and language activities. Without a Statement such additional time may be at the expense of other activities and will be very much at the discretion of school staff. However the time is arranged it is important that it can be used as effectively and efficiently as possible. This means that any programme must be easy to implement and the materials must be readily available (see Figures 6.3 and 6.4). With the introduction of literacy and numeracy hours in September 1998, coordination of other activities may become increasingly difficult.

### Staff training

Teachers may be involved in a range of both school-based and external in-service training. It is now quite common for speech and language clinicians to run training courses for special needs assistants, special needs coordinators and other interested staff. This is seen as a way of providing information, as well as changing attitudes and building good working relationships. The survey by Jowett and Evans (1996) found that although these were well received, there were difficulties when LEAs were expected to fund such training. However, uptake of places was high when the training was seen to be free.

School staff also have a commitment to attending a set number of staff development sessions during the year. Many schools will run in-service training (INSET) days, where the speech and language clinician may contribute either as presenter or participant. Other training may take place through ongoing involvement with staff in the classroom setting. Involvement in these situations can also give the speech and language clinician greater understanding of current educational issues and school policies, as well as building on their relationship with the school staff.

Some LEAs are now organizing more formal training for special needs/classroom assistants, and various health professionals may be invited to contribute to these courses.

| A programme should include: |
|---|
| **Summary of present skills** This can be used to highlight current or newly acquired skills as a foundation for the present aims |
| **Clear aims** These should be written in easily understandable language that relate to activities already going on in the classroom. For example, if the class is covering a particular science topic, make sure that the programme is focusing on the same vocabulary and concepts |
| **Context** It may be helpful to specify the setting in which activities should take place, i.e. group, quiet corner, etc. |
| **Materials needed** If you are not able to supply these, make sure the assistant has a full list of everything that will be needed before the activity is begun. It may be useful to have them collected together in a clearly labelled box or corner |
| **Procedures/suggested activities** You will need to provide a range of activities for each aim, so that there is variety for both the child and the assistant |
| **Reinforcement/feedback** How should this be incorporated into the activity? It needs to be simple and relevant so that it is done on a routine basis |
| **Record keeping** This needs to be a quick and easily managed process, which documents the input and progress of the child |
| **General considerations** This would include suggestions for how to encourage carry-over of new skills into other contexts |
| **Review** What should be done in case of difficulties? How can you be contacted? It should also include an indication of when the programme will be reviewed |

**Figure 6.3:** Guidelines for writing a programme.

### Input into school policies and curriculum development

Finally, speech and language clinicians can be seen as a resource in relation to speech and language development. They may be able to contribute to more general aspects of the language curriculum, and in particular the speaking and listening components of the National Curriculum and the Literacy hour. Speech and language clinicians should make themselves aware of the policies in operation in the schools in which they are working. This may include policies on:

- language and literacy
- child protection
- dealing with challenging behaviour.

NAME: Lisa M.                      D.O.B: 8/8/92          C.A: 6:1

SCHOOL: Whitegates Special School       DATE: 12/9/98

Summary of present communication
Lisa is beginning to use language appropriately but needs to extend her organization of language and language concepts

Aims of programme
1. To develop her understanding of instructions containing four information-
carrying words, e.g. 'Give the little cow a big cup'.
2. To develop her ability to give instructions containing three elements, e.g. 'Put the
car under the table'

Context
Lisa is easily distracted, so it will help her to work in a quiet distraction-free environment

Materials needed
1. A set of large and small everyday objects and a large and small box and bag
2. Large and small dolls and teddies
3. Symbol pictures
4. Farmyard picture, and two sets of identical farm animals

Suggested activities
1. Give L. instructions about where to put the objects away, e.g. 'Put the big spoon in
the big box'. Take it in turns so L. then asks you to put something away, using the
name of the object and its location. Try to discourage her from just pointing. When
she is giving you instructions you may need to simplify it so she only labels the
object rather that thinking about the size, e.g. 'Put the spoon in the big bag'

2. Direct L. to carry out a range of actions, e.g. 'Wash the big teddy's feet', 'Put little
teddy under the table'. Again try role reversal so she then gives you directions as to
what she wants

3. Take it in turns to colour in the symbol pictures, e.g. 'Make the little pig red'

4. Try a barrier-type game involving another child, where you use a screen or box so
you can't see what each other has done. Set the animals around the farm for L. She
has to tell the other child what to do to make hers the same, e.g. 'The cow is next to
the house, the duck is on the pond'. Then change them over so that the other child
gives the directions to L. The adult will need to help to make sure they do this orally,
rather than by pointing

If L. enjoys this type of activity I'm sure you will come up with lots of other ideas

Reinforcement/feedback
L. should find most of these activities rewarding in their own right, but remember to
give her verbal encouragement and model the correct response if she is having difficulty

**Figure 6.4:** Example of a programme.                               (contd)

Record-keeping
Please can you complete the attached form to give me feedback on the activities

General considerations
Once L. is feeling confident with these types of tasks it may be helpful to incorporate them into 'circle time' with the whole class group

Review
This programme will be reviewed again in January 1999, but please contact me before then if you require any further ideas or support

Signed

**Figure 6.4:** (contd)

## Personnel

### *The headteacher*

It should be remembered that the head is in overall charge of the school and should be kept informed of your contact with the children in the school. They are 'in loco parentis' and therefore ultimately responsible for the child while he or she is on the school premises.

### *The special educational needs coordinator (SENCO)*

Each school should have an appointed SENCO who has responsibility for implementing the school's special educational needs policy and monitoring children on the Special Needs Register. He or she will also be involved in supporting staff with the assessment process and providing teaching support. His or her role will also be to liaise with external professionals. In many cases the SENCO may be the main point of contact for the speech and language clinician.

### *The child protection coordinator*

Schools should also have an appointed member of staff with responsibility for child protection issues. This person should be your first point of contact if you have any concerns about a child who you feel may have suffered some form of abuse. He or she is responsible for contact with outside agencies while the child is at school.

### *The special needs assistant*

Some children may have a full- or part-time assistant appointed as part of their Statement of Educational Need. Assistants will have a clearly defined role within the classroom in relation to this child, and this may include speech and language therapy support. Other assistants may be appointed to support a group or class of children, but may be able to follow up on speech and language programmes.

### The class teacher

Although initial contact may be made through the special needs coordinator, it is important to remember that the class teacher is responsible for the day-to-day management of the child and should be kept involved with the speech and language programme. The availability of the child, work in the classroom, etc., should be negotiated directly with the class teacher.

### The school nurse

Some special schools, especially those catering for children with physical disabilities, may have a full-time school nurse who will be responsible for medication and health care. All main stream schools will have a designated school nurse who may cover several schools in the area. The nurse can be a useful source of information and can arrange medical checks on request.

### The clinical medical officer

This is a doctor employed by the health authority, whose job is to oversee the health needs of the school population. He or she is likely to conduct medicals on children as part of the statementing process, and is responsible for coordinating all the advice from the health professionals.

### The advisory teacher

LEAs may employ a number of advisory teachers to provide support to schools in the area. This support is usually provided to the teaching staff in terms of resources and advice, but may also involve direct interaction with the child. Advisory teachers may include specialist teachers for visually impaired children, hearing impaired children, information technology, etc.

### The educational psychologist

The educational psychologist will have a key role to play in the decision-making process and in many cases will be responsible for the coordination of the formal statementing process. He or she will also give advice to teachers on educational and behavioural management.

## Work with social welfare personnel

Speech and language clinicians may work in a range of settings that are organized and funded by the local authority social services department.

They may also liaise with fieldwork social workers in relation to specific clients in their care.

## Residential settings and day services

## The elderly and disabled

### Residential care

Residential care (Table 6.2), commonly referred to as 'Part III accommodation', should be provided for anyone over the age of 18 who needs it because of age, disability or illness. This does not involve any level of medical care. However, since the introduction of the NHS and Community Care Act (1990) much of this care is now provided by the private sector and is the result of a full assessment of need. Some facilities are still run by social services and they remain responsible for the overall inspection and approval of residential services. Some district or trust policies do not provide for therapy input into such homes. Other managers argue that the residential establishment is the client's home and so they should be provided with the same domiciliary support as those people still residing within their own homes.

As well as working with individual clients in this setting, the speech and language clinician may organize group therapy, such as setting up 'Reminiscence Groups'. They may also advise on how to maintain and create an environment to promote effective communication between residents.

**Table 6.2:** Residential care

|                     | Acute emergency care | Rehabilitation/continuing care |
|---------------------|----------------------|--------------------------------|
| Home-based          | Intensive home support<br>Emergency duty teams<br>Sector teams | Domiciliary services<br>Key workers<br>Care management |
| Day care            | Day hospitals        | Drop-in centres<br>Support groups<br>Employment schemes<br>Day care |
| Residential support | Crisis accommodation<br>Acute units<br>Local secure units | Ordinary housing<br>Unstaffed group homes<br>Adult placement schemes<br>Residential care homes<br>Mental nursing homes<br>24-hour NHS accommodation<br>Medium secure units<br>High security units |

DoH (1993: 71).

*Day centres*

Services are also being provided in day centres, which may be totally funded by social services or a joint initiative with health trusts. Here the speech and language clinician may work with both individuals and groups. There may also be staff available to do follow-up work with clients.

*Domiciliary care*

Social services may provide staffed support to enable clients to stay in their own home rather than requiring residential care. The provision of this service is means tested, and it will be closely linked to informal care provided by friends and relatives. Help may be given for shopping, house-work and personal care, including provision of some meals and help with bathing, dressing, etc. The home care worker is a vital link between the client and other services and can provide support as well as monitoring changes in the client's health and wellbeing.

*Care management*

Where the needs of a client are complex or involve significant resources, the social services department will need to arrange for an assessment of need. The care manager will arrange for this assessment and help to draw up a care plan. The role of the care manager is then to purchase the resources and services outlined in the plan and to monitor and review its implementation; they are not responsible for the provision of these services. Care may be purchased from a range of statutory and voluntary and private agencies.

The core tasks of care management are:

1. publication of information about what resources are available
2. determining the level of assessment needed
3. assessing need
4. care planning
5. implementing the care plan
6. monitoring
7. reviewing.

**Adults with learning disabilities**

The concept of 'normalization' or 'social role valorization' emerged from the USA in the 1970s and has significantly altered attitudes and provision for adults with learning disabilities. Increasingly they are being moved from long-stay institutions to small group settings within the community. Foxen and McBrien (1981) describe five key values for a service promoting 'ordinary life' values:

1. Community presence: both residential and day services within the community.
2. Competence: the development of skills in order to participate in the local community.
3. Choice: promotion of a range of options and opportunities.
4. Respect: service should help people to enjoy the same status as other valued members of society.
5. Relationships: service should help and encourage individuals to mix with other non-disabled people.

With this move into the community has come the need to develop appropriate communication skills to enable effective participation in community life. As a part of care management these clients will have an individual assessment leading to an Individual Programme Plan (IPP). These plans are written in collaboration with the client and carers, and reflect their needs and wishes for the future. Increasingly, speech and language intervention is being included in these plans and there has been a significant development in services for this client group.

*Individual programme planning*

A coordinator will usually be appointed to support the client and collect together information which will be presented at the IPP meeting. This information will focus on the client's strengths and needs.
  Areas considered may include:

- basic physical skills
- communication skills
- self-care and domestic skills
- recreation and leisure skills and opportunities
- social skills and personal relationships
- medical and financial needs.

At the meeting this information will be considered, and a plan of goals agreed with the client will be drawn up. Clear decisions will be made and documented about who will take responsibility for each part of this programme. This plan will be reviewed as part of subsequent annual IPP meetings.

*Supported living/group homes*

This move to the community has involved considerable changes in the philosophy and working practices of staff involved. The speech and language clinician must be able to respond in a flexible manner to the training needs of staff as well as the therapy needs of the clients. However, it should be remembered that most adults with learning disabilities continue to live with their family, who may also require a range of different kinds of help and support.

*Day care provision*

*Social education centres/adult training centres*

Traditionally, Adult Training Centres were set up to provide sheltered employment for adults with learning disabilities living in the community. More recently these have become social education centres, where there is an emphasis on continuing education and the development of the skills needed to live successfully within the community. Here the speech and language clinician may work with individual clients and groups of clients and may also be involved with staff development and training. The client's time at the centre may be integrated with a range of other activities in the community, including part-time attendance at a college and work experience. Any intervention will need to be carefully coordinated and based on the current and future needs of the client.

*Further education*

In recent years there has been a growth in the number of courses catering for this client group. This may be a specific full-time course designed to help with the transition from school to adult life, or clients may access a range of individual adult education classes. These may include academic skills, such as literacy and numeracy, or may provide access to leisure activities.

*Clients with mental health problems*

Social services departments may coordinate a range of services for people with mental health problems. They will harness resources provided by statutory agencies, the voluntary and private sectors. Reforms in the early 1990s set out to see more services being contracted out by social service departments to the voluntary and private sectors.

**Children**

The Children Act 1989 outlines the provision that should be made for the care of children. Although in exceptional circumstances a court order can be made to take the child into residential care, wherever possible every effort is made to keep the child in their family home. The Act states that a decision to remove the child from the home must only be made if it is in the best interests of the child. Links should be maintained with the family if at all possible.

*Residential care*

Social services will provide residential care:
1. *Foster homes* If possible the child will be placed within a family network of specially recruited and trained foster parents. They will have undergone a careful selection process and will be supported by a social work team. They will be involved with all aspects of the child's life and will be encouraged to build links with the child's natural family. They will also be responsible for keeping medical appointments and will be encouraged to work closely with all professionals involved with the child.
2. *Respite care* This may be provided for children with disabilities which may cause strain on the family. Respite care for a night, weekend or short break may be provided by specially recruited respite foster parents or through a staffed hostel. The speech and language clinician may need to give advice and training to respite carers to ensure a consistent approach to the development of communication and feeding skills.
3. *Group homes* These provide secure accommodation for children whose behaviour has made it difficult for them to remain within the family home. Specially trained staff will develop programmes and provide appropriate supervision.

*Day care*

1. *Family centres/day nurseries* These centres provide support for families of pre-school children. They may provide nursery care for children from the age of 3 months onwards, but will also support and work with parents. Some nursery places will be made available for children who require social service supervision because of suspected abuse or neglect, and others may provide special facilities for children with disabilities. The centre will be managed by a qualified nursery nurse or teacher and will be staffed by qualified nursery nurses. Some centres may also run after-school clubs. In some areas the speech and language clinician may work within the nursery setting on a regular basis. Staff may be willing to carry out programmes left by the speech and language clinician or help with running language groups or sessions with parents.
2. *Play schemes* Many local authorities will run play schemes in the school holidays to provide a safe and stimulating environment for children. Special play schemes may be organized for children with disabilities.

# Fieldwork

As well as a range of day and residential services, social services departments will have staff who will be involved with clients on an individual basis. The fieldwork social worker may be involved with:

- visiting families of children at risk of abuse/neglect
- supervision of children protected by a court order
- supervision of children for adoption and fostering
- statutory duties in relation to people with a mental illness who require compulsory care or compulsory hospitalization
- support and advice to all client groups and their carers
- specialist services, for example to the blind, deaf, etc.
- provision of a hospital social work service.

The speech and language clinician may need to liaise directly with an individual social worker about the needs of a client, for example in relation to discharge from hospital, financial hardship, etc. At other times they may be involved in a more formal way, such as in relation to child protection. Here they may be part of a large team of professionals involved with a particular child and their family.

### Child protection

The child protection services will consist of a multidisciplinary team involving health, education, the police and the National Society for the Prevention of Cruelty to Children (NSPCC). The social services department will be the lead agency and will take responsibility for the service and for maintenance of the Child Protection Register. It is important that all speech and language clinicians working with children attend local training in child protection so that they are familiar with local policies and procedures. This includes how to gain information about children on the Child Protection Register, as well as the procedures to follow if abuse or neglect is alleged or suspected (see Figure 6.5).

The speech and language clinician may be aware of general or specific communication behaviours that could be indicative of abuse or neglect. It is important that this information is clearly documented and the clinician is prepared to give evidence in court.

### Personnel

#### Care manager

He/she is not involved in direct service delivery. He or she will arrange for the client to have an assessment of need and is then responsible for the design and implementation of care to meet this need.

#### Home care worker

He/she may perform a range of tasks to enable the client to remain in their home environment.

#### Key worker

He/she usually carries the main service-providing role and is responsible

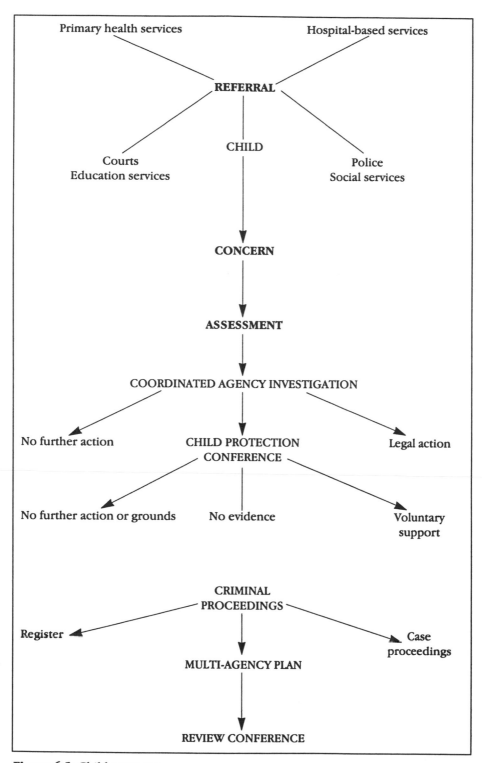

**Figure 6.5**: Child protection process.

for coordinating the involvement of all professionals working with the client. Provides a central point for communication.

*Field worker*

He/she will be appointed to a client or family to give support and advice.

*Occupational therapist*

Some occupational therapists will be employed by social services departments. They play an important role in the assessment and support of people with a disability.

*Specialist social worker*

Some departments will employ social workers who have specialist knowledge in relation to particular client groups, for example deaf people, and clients with visual impairment.

*Duty social worker*

Social service departments will always have a member of staff on call in an emergency. This duty social worker may deal with a crisis and then hand the client on to other staff in the department.

# Working with volunteers and the private sector

There are an increasing number of voluntary and private institutions and agencies providing health and social care to clients. Recent reorganization of social service provision has encouraged a range of agencies to be involved in contributing a package of care.

## Working with volunteers and in voluntary agencies

The speech and language clinician may also be involved with supervising volunteers in the work setting. These may be an extremely valuable resource. However, some of the considerations discussed in relation to working with assistants may also be applicable here. There are also other issues that need to be considered.

There should be a careful system of selection and screening of potential volunteers. It is important to check procedures with your own personnel department as there are likely to be insurance implications, and there may be a requirement for police and health checks to be carried out. It is also important that the role and contribution of the volunteer is clearly defined before their involvement starts, and that his or her work is supervised closely. Clients should be consulted about the volunteer's role, and consent to their involvement should be gained. Some of the differences between an assistant employed by the department and a volunteer are given in Table 6.3.

Table 6.3: Some differences between an assistant and a volunteer

| Assistant | Volunteer |
| --- | --- |
| Full/part time- involved in range of aspects of therapy | Usually involved with one client-specific task |
| Obliged to keep records | No compulsion to keep records |
| Formal supervision essential | May not receive regular supervision |
| Work usually in formal setting – clinic, school, hospital | May work in clinic, hospital, school and client's home |
| Has job description, standards, disciplinary procedures | Has negotiated role, choice and freedom |
| Personnel responsible for: | Need careful vetting for: |
|    health checks |    health checks |
|    police checks, etc. |    police checks, etc. |

## Charitable organizations

Several charitable organizations employ their own speech and language clinicians. These agencies are usually involved in the provision of specialist care and advice for a particular client group. For example:

- SCOPE provides information, assessment and educational and social care for children and adults with cerebral palsy.
- Action for Dysphasic Adults (ADA) provides an information and advice service for speech and language clinicians, relatives of people with aphasia and others involved in their care.
- The Motor Neurone Disease Association provides specialist advice and support to sufferers and their families.
- The Honourmead Trust runs several schools for children with learning disabilities, specific language impairment, etc.
- ICAN (Invalid Children's Association Nationwide) is responsible for several residential schools for children with specific language impairment.

There are certain advantages for the clinician working in these types of settings. Probably the most important is the chance to gain specialist experience with a particular client group, and the opportunity to work alongside staff who are specialists in the field. There may also be a significantly reduced caseload in comparison with clinicians working for a statutory agency. In some instances these charities may have greater resources for equipment and additional staff training, but this is certainly not always the case.

On the other hand, in a small organization there may be little opportunity for contact with other speech and language clinicians. The management structure may mean that supervision is provided by someone from a different clinical background who may not fully understand the role of the speech and language clinician. There are also issues such as pay and conditions and pension arrangements that may be less clearly negotiated and defined prior to taking up the post.

Advantages include:

• experience with a specialist client group, often with specialist support
• increased autonomy and the possibility to shape your own role
• a smaller case load
• improved resources and access to training.

Disadvantages include:

• professional isolation, because of small number employed
• isolation from broader speech and language context and developments
• organizational structure may mean that manager is not a speech and language clinician
• lack of recognition of experience when returning to more traditional employment
• differences in conditions of service, e.g. superannuation, holiday entitlement, etc.

## The private sector

### *Private health care and private hospitals*

In the UK, speech and language therapy is frequently not covered by private medical insurance. The provision of therapy services in private hospitals and care homes is usually on an individual basis and provided by a speech and language clinician in private practice.

### *Private practice*

There has been a steady increase in the numbers of speech and language clinicians being employed in the private sector or choosing to be independent practitioners. The RCSLT recommends that clinicians should have a minimum of two years' experience before venturing into private practice. There is now an Association of Speech and Language Therapists in Independent Practice (ASTIIP) which is affiliated to the RCSLT. The RCSLT also gives clear guidelines about liaison with therapists within the private sector. These include:

• the primacy of client care rests with the NHS therapist if care is being shared with an independent practitioner
• the lead role in coordination of care normally rests with the NHS therapist

- if a client opts for private therapy while on a waiting list for NHS treatment, their name should remain on the waiting list unless the client specifically asks for its removal
- an NHS therapist should not disclose any information to a private therapist without the written consent of the client/carer involved.

For further information see RCSLT (1996: 310).

Anybody interested in working in the private sector in Great Britain must be registered as a private practitioner with the RCSLT and should contact ASTIIP for advice. Clients enquiring about private therapy should be encouraged to discuss this with their GP or contact ASTIIP. A speech and language therapist employed by a statutory agency should not provide private therapy for any of the clients on their caseload. They should provide the client with information about how to contact a suitably qualified therapist.

**Locum agencies**

There are an increasing number of locum agencies who are prepared to put speech and language clinicians on their books. Although some of them will consider including newly qualified therapists on their list, it is recommended that the clinician should have had some generalized experience and have gained full clinical autonomy in a supervised setting.

These agencies may be contacted by statutory bodies or charitable/ private institutions who wish to fill employment gaps. The agency will provide potential employers with details of their charges and details of a number of clinicians who may fit the job criteria. The employer will want up-to-date information about experience, along with references from past employers and other agency experience. Any contract is likely to be short-term because this is an expensive way for employers to fill vacancies.

# Summary

The development of team-working and the coordinated care of clients can be of significant benefit to the client, the family and the professionals involved. However, team-working is not an easy option, and it requires careful consideration, planning and commitment from all professionals and agencies involved. There is also a need for evaluation and audit of such enterprises so that we can become clearer about what the benefits might be. Also we need to identify the factors and influences that go towards creating and maintaining an effective team.

However, it must always be remembered that the key player in this team is the client. Clients' needs and wishes must be seen as paramount in the decision-making process.

# Chapter 7
# Record keeping and Reporting

One of the cries heard from some clinicians is 'If only there were not so much paper work ... all these records, reports, letters, statements and statistics ... it keeps me away from the real work.'

Let us think this through in a more positive way. We should never underestimate how much written communications, records and data collection are a part of the real work. The paperwork, that is the information systems of records and reports, is a very significant aspect of client management and the provision of an effective and efficient service.

- Without records and reports where is the accurate documentation of our knowledge of the client, the assessments we have used, the intervention we have given, the contacts with and contributions of other personnel, the responses of the client, and the progress that has taken place?
- Without records and reports how do other personnel know precisely what has taken place or become familiar with what the service provides?
- Without records and reports how can the work of the speech and language service be objectively evaluated for effectiveness and resource needs?

Recording and reporting must be viewed not as arduous or unnecessary evils, but as integral to the delivery of speech and language services to clients, and must be respected for the role they have in providing a formal mechanism for speech and language professional accountability.

This chapter will in particular look at three forms of information systems that have a significant place in speech and language therapy clinical practice: case records, reports and statistics. The aim is to:

1. provide an understanding of the purposes of information systems
2. consider some of the legal and ethical implications of information systems

3. offer guidelines for good practice in the compilation of information systems.

# Case records

Case records constitute a formal record of information pertinent to the speech and language management of a particular client. As a speech and language clinician you are responsible for any entry you have made and hence legally and professionally accountable for what is written. While a speech and language case record, or file, will be kept for each client from the date of referral and retained even after discharge, this is not necessarily the sole record of speech and language management for which you will be responsible. Dependent on the clinical context you may need to contribute with a range of personnel to other types of case records. Two examples of these, medical records and care plans, are explained below, in addition to the discussion of speech and language case records.

### Medical records

For clients who are hospital inpatients the medical records kept on the ward are key in communications between the professionals involved, and facilitate the day-to-day multidisciplinary coordination of information about contacts made, assessment findings, diagnosis, intervention, progress and recommendations. Entries in the notes by the speech and language clinician are a professional obligation. These must be relevant and brief, respecting that no one has time to read more than the bare essentials and remembering that communication about the client is not restricted to the highlights you include here. You will also be using other communication channels, such as ward rounds, case conferences and meetings with specific professionals, as well as written reports and regular entries in the ward Cardex system, to share information and guide the decision-making process.

In the medical records a very few words can be used for example:

1. To confirm that you have responded to a referral, made an initial contact, identified significant problems or an initial diagnosis, and to indicate your immediate intentions and recommendations:

   Drowsy, confused; language comprehension severely impaired; speech output restricted to unintelligible jargon; motor skills unaffected in feeding and speech. To further assess. (Your signature and the date)

2. To give information about change, family contact and advice given, and indicate future plans:

   Depressed, deterioration in swallowing function, speech no longer a viable means of communication. Patient and wife advised on alternative communication methods. Appointment with Communication Aids Centre arranged. To continue to see after imminent discharge home. (Your signature and the date)

## Care plans

It is commonly a care management plan, which is a contract of care provision, that enables the delivery of a coordinated package of care for a person. These might be used for a child or an adult with multiple disabilities or with learning difficulties, who has a range of identified needs. This statement of needs places care within a functional and social context. A care plan might be drawn up for a person living in his or her own or family home, or for a person living in a residential centre or community home. In either case the individual may or may not attend a rehabilitation or development unit, or a day or education centre. Initially, a functional assessment of the needs of the individual would be made. Then the multidisciplinary team, in conjunction with the client and, where appropriate, his or her next of kin, guardian or advocate, would negotiate a care management plan, which specifies objectives for care and identifies the personnel responsible for providing appropriate support to meet these objectives. In this way, qualified and unqualified personnel from a range of health and social care agencies (e.g. physiotherapists, home care assistants, residential care assistants, district nurses, nursing assistants, occupational therapists, social workers, and speech and language therapists) have a common point of reference, enabling them to record and share understandings about the physical, functional and social needs of the individual, and determine the extent to which the objectives of the care management plan have been met.

*Communication* is one of the categories that may be included in the care plan, and for which the speech and language clinician may have direct or indirect responsibility. If this is the case the clinician would negotiate and agree specific objectives relating to speech and language and swallowing function, record progress and recommend any modifications required in the light of change. Once more we have an information system that contains a record of evidence from a range of personnel involved in the care of the client, which will be readily available to everyone. To be effective in contributing to the care of the individual, all entries must be concise and written in language that will be accessible to everyone, including professionals from a range of disciplines and non-professional care givers. Additionally as with any other record, entries must be dated and signed, and hence owned by the author.

Figure 7.1 gives an example of an extract from a care plan showing how the speech and language clinician contributes to the record.

## Speech and language case records

The speech and language case record constitutes a file of all the data relating to the client who has been referred to the speech and language clinician. This is not merely a device to remind us about the client from week to week, but a comprehensive account that will be passed on to

(date)
1.  To locate 4 additional Blissymbols on request – garden, bird, flower, tree.
2.  To spontaneously use symbols in social speech – e.g. hello, fine, hungry.
3.  To initiate 2 symbol questions – e.g. where nurse? when mum (coming)? what weather (like)?

Recommendations:
    Practise location of new and previously introduced symbols.
    Engage him in social speech question and answer.
    Encourage him to ask you questions.
    (your signature)

**Figure 7.1:** How the speech and language clinician contributes to the record.

other speech and language clinicians who may be involved in the management of the client at a later date. It is also the account that serves as the reference point for any issues relating to the case that arise during the current episode of care or in the future, even after discharge from speech and language intervention, and up to the death of the client. Hence, it is vital that as new information is known it is recorded. Even if you think you can remember, the details will fade or distort over time, and they will not have been made available to others unless they are written down as soon as possible.

The contents of the case record file will vary. In the case of a person who was seen for initial assessment only, there may be little more than the essential client details, a minimal note of referral and background information, the assessment findings and conclusions from the meeting with the client, and a copy of the discharge report. Another person might have a more long-standing and complex history of contact with speech and language clinicians, which could result in a rather weighty case record. Further, each speech and language service will have a different framework for the record. None the less it is helpful to outline the components that will normally be included in the case record:

*   client identification data
*   diagnosis
*   background details
*   presenting problems
*   intervention.

### Client identification data

This includes the name, date of birth, sex, address, telephone number, hospital number (if applicable), referring agent details, date of referral, GP details, school (if applicable) and next of kin. It is important to also make a note of the reason for referral, the date of the initial appointment and, when the time arrives, the date of discharge, with a note of the reason for discharge (e.g. death, transfer to another authority, mutual agreement with the client or non-attendance). As the discussion of statistics described below explains, some of this information will be translated into codes for data collection and analysis.

Thus clinicians make sure that they have all the data they need to identify each client both in their written communications and for statistical records, and to facilitate their basic communications with and about the client.

*Diagnosis*

This constitutes the speech and language diagnosis made by you, the expert in speech and language pathology, for example 'delayed phonological disorder'; 'semantic-pragmatic disorder'; 'cluttering'. Additionally it is often helpful to include a reference to any significant aetiological factors that explain the nature of the disorder, for example 'hearing impairment'; 'auditory attention deficit'; 'cerebral vascular accident'; 'no known causation'.

The final diagnosis of the communication disorder may be difficult to ascertain until some time has passed and a full picture of the problem(s) has evolved from the data collection, hypothesis formulation and hypothesis testing process of assessment. Only when this point is reached are you in a position to confirm a diagnosis. However, you do need to provide at least a broad and tentative diagnosis at an early stage for the purposes of communication and statistical records. Hence it is not uncommon for the case file to have two headings: 'Provisional diagnosis', to be completed at first contact, and 'Diagnosis', to be completed as soon as a differential diagnosis of the communication disorder has been made. Thus the provisional diagnoses of 'non-fluency', 'moderate dysarthria' and 'speech disorder', which describe three different individuals after the first contact, may be rewritten in the course of time as diagnoses of 'severe stammering', 'moderately severe progressive mixed spastic and flaccid dysarthria (due to motor neurone disease)' and 'developmental expressive language and articulatory disorder (due to cleft palate)'.

*Background details*

This includes all the case history details, as well as additional information about the client that will emerge in the course of contact with him or her. The client's background will be learned from a range of data-collection procedures, discussed in Chapter 3 (e.g. case history taken from the client and/or carer; medical notes; school reports; ongoing information from the client, family, friends and other carers and personnel who are in contact with the client). When recording information in the file, it is important to provide dates to ensure that there is a chronological record of events. Additionally you should note sources of information whenever possible so that discrepancies can be identified and evaluated. For example, a mother might report her child had normal hearing, but an audiogram might indicate a reduction in acuity in certain frequencies that would be of minimal concern for most children, but in conjunction with a range of factors presenting in a particular child could be significant.

Case files generally contain sections for key aspects of background details within which we can add information as it emerges. 'Medical', 'Personal and social' and 'Development' are common headings; however, these will obviously differ depending on the client group. The sections are likely to be guided according to the varying information we need to record for acquired, adult, developmental or child disorders.

## Presenting problems

It is always important to have a record of the disorder as it presented at the first contact with a speech and language clinician. This serves as the baseline for your future investigations and as a reference point for your evaluation of progress. Clinicians should record a description of the presenting features of the impairment, indicating the strengths and weaknesses and influences on communication function they observe.

For example:

- Gait unsteady, clinging to mother for most of session, unable to complete simple form-board; responded to name, able to identify familiar pictured items from name; follows two idea commands 50%; speech restricted to monosyllabic utterances not identifiable as words, consonants fronted.
- Good concentration and insight into communication difficulty; anxious that will be unable to return to previous employment. Comprehension 100% in social level conversation. Western Aphasia Battery: auditory verbal comprehension – 57/60, yes/no questions – 60/60, auditory word recognition/sequential commands – 70/80. Reading comprehension delayed but accurate at level of short simple paragraph. Speech output non-fluent where increased demand for specific content. Word retrieval problems characterized by semantic paraphasia and repair, aided by phonemic cues and semantic associations. Agrammatic due to limited use of function words and appropriate word endings. Moderate intelligibility; able to communicate messages with some success but linguistic accuracy impaired. Spontaneous writing from picture stimulus not possible. Writing to dictation of common words legible, but only accurate in spelling simple short words with regular spellings.

*Intervention*

This will include a record of dates and findings of formal and informal assessments, copies of which (e.g. samples of speech, drawings and writing, as well as completed assessment record sheets from published or clinician designed assessments) may be included as an appendix to the case file to provide evidence of performance and progress. Additionally, this will contain a record of direct and indirect intervention, written in a clear but very concise style making sure the objectives and outcomes are identified. Where evidence is available, such as letters and reports to and from other professionals, these should also be included in chronological order in a separate section of the file.

The main body of the case record or file will be in the form of chronologically dated and signed entries. These may consist of a record of a telephone call made or received concerning the client, the conclusions of a conversation with a teacher, or a summary of a session with the client. Also objective-based management decisions and recommendations as well as evidence of change will be noted at relevant places within the ongoing account.

It is not uncommon to have concerns about the style and acceptable content when making entries in the case file. While each clinician will develop a somewhat idiosyncratic manner there are golden rules that must be followed in order to meet your legal and professional obligations.

The account should be:

- accurate
- comprehensive
- contemporaneous, i.e. written as soon as possible after the contact, anything more than 24 hours after the event has reduced validity and credibility
- legible
- relevant
- signed.

If you have planned your intervention thoroughly with clearly defined objectives, the account should be quite easy to write.

1. Remember to use unambiguous, concise language.
2. Indicate assessment findings and the objective for each aspect of therapy and the outcomes achieved by the client.
3. Note any observations or additional information that emerged during the contact.
4. State both action you have taken and recommendations you propose.
5. Date and sign the entry.

Below are two examples, one of good and one of bad practice, of case report entries written following a session with a 4-year-old boy with severe language comprehension problems.

1. Jamie arrived in a new jersey today, played happily with the cars but could not indicate the colours when asked. Would sometimes not give me the toys in the order I requested. Did not say very much today. Looked unhappy but would not say what was wrong. Apparently has been in trouble at the nursery this morning. I asked Mrs P if I could see Jamie at home next week, which she agreed.
2. Small toy play age appropriate.
   Colour concept (red and blue) development: (a) Cars sorted by colour (red/blue) 100%; (b) auditory verbal comprehension of colour names 20%; (c) imitation of the colour name for the red items sorted encouraged to develop word association, achieved for all items.
   Auditory verbal memory: Identification of familiar monosyllabic nouns (spoon, doll, car and ball) by name 100%. Memory for the nouns 100% for two items, 70% correct for three items and 30% for four items.
   Reserved behaviour with episodes of lapses in attention. Did not initiate conversation.
   Mother reports his difficulty in following instructions at nursery, and slowness to respond results in the other children teasing him. Agreed to contact nursery.
   Home visit arranged for next week to evaluate communication in familiar environment.                                            (signed and dated)

You can see from the second example that:

- there is no need to include either the name of the child, nor mention yourself, this can be taken as known
- subjective comments (e.g. 'looks', 'seems', 'appears') must be avoided, only facts are of interest
- wherever possible, measurements should be included; from this, performance and change can be accurately conveyed
- management decisions should be clearly indicated.
- entries must be signed and dated.

A well-written entry will:

- facilitate the delivery of service to the client
- provide documentary evidence of the service delivered
- facilitate the continuity of care
- discharge a contractual duty to the employer
- contribute to the preparation of reports and statements
- assist the mechanism of accountability
- contribute to the evaluation of the service offered (RCSLT, 1996).

*Defensible documentation*

Although the professional and legal status of the case records has been emphasized, this should be explained in context and with further detail to support the clinician in recording information.

The case record is a defensible document. This means that it constitutes primary evidence, i.e. original documentation, and as such can be used in litigation cases. A demand for the submission of case records for use as evidence may be made in rare instances when the management of a client by the speech and language therapy service has been questioned. More commonly the records are required to contribute to cases of alleged medical negligence, compensation agreements, or in family or criminal cases in which the communication disorder is perceived to be a factor. This provides a further reason for the requirement to retain any record that is written during the life of an individual. Even if a record is damaged, whether by tearing or tea spillage, for legal purposes it must be retained in this state.

Professional opinion expressed on any personal health records, and this includes speech and language therapy records, remains the property of the author. It is essential to confirm authorship at the time of writing by adding the date and your normal signature, not merely by initialling the account. You should be confident that what is written is accurate, unambiguous, sufficiently detailed and legible. The author is responsible for whatever is written and so has to be prepared to defend the account if required.

Since clinicians have such responsibility for what they write, they must ensure that there is no doubt about the detail and authenticity of what is included, and that it will stand up in court if necessary. First, anything written should not be altered by obliterating the original entry. Instead you must put a single line through the error and date and initial the change. Second, if abbreviations are used make sure a key is supplied so that they can be understood by other personnel.

In Britain, since the Access to Health Records Act of 1990, clients have had a right to access all personal information held on both manual (written) and computerized health records. The proviso is that access can be withheld if the information is deemed likely to cause them or another person physical or mental harm. This is particularly the case where the records include information about another individual who might be identified if access were given. Knowing that the client can make a request and in the majority of cases can see their records, reminds us of the importance of including objective and clear details. It is considered professionally unacceptable to record trivia or pejorative remarks, but knowing that your notes can be seen outside your own tight professional circle certainly helps focus your style.

*Computer and joint records*

So far this overview of case records has concentrated on manual systems of record keeping. In recent years, with a view to a wide range of knowledge about their clients being readily available to every professional involved in their care, computerized and joint case recording systems have been introduced in some health services. This requires a dedication to confidentiality and security of passwords so that entry to the system and information held is confined to authorized personnel. Additionally, practical problems may need to be overcome. For example: having access to a computer to input data as soon as possible after contact or other intervention; the technical skills of the clinician in receiving and inputting data; the ability of the system to cope with such things as phonetic symbols; and including data that have uniformity with those of other users. However, the use of computerized systems certainly increases the chance of professionals becoming conversant with each other's management decisions and makes information sharing more open and more speedy. In effect it should contribute to improved client care.

Records of all types are also valuable sources of data for research and audit. Not only do records form an integral part of the management of the individual client, but they can contribute to wider contexts, such as the constant search for new understandings of communication disorders and their mangement and the endeavour to ensure that service provision is of the highest quality.

## Case reports

It is not uncommon for the inexperienced clinician to have concerns about report writing, such as how to know when to send a report, what it should contain, how long and detailed it should be, the style in which it should be written and to whom copies should be sent. Most of these anxieties will become insignificant as you gain greater familiarity with the codes of practice of your own professional organization and the standards and practices of the individual speech and language service where you are working, as you are exposed to examples of reports received or sent by other speech and language clinicians and as your experience of actual report writing increases. Here we will offer a few general comments on some of the practical issues involved.

Broad guidance concerning report writing is provided by the Royal College of Speech and Language Therapists (RCSLT, 1996), which identifies three types of reports defined by different stages of overall management. These are:

1. an initial report following assessment
2. an interim report as and when necessary following referral
3. a closure report following discharge.

Local guidelines and the standards of practice of your speech and language therapy service are likely to provide more detailed information about when and how to report. In the case of interim reports, much will depend on your own judgement and on the requirements of other agencies. You are likely to report if you have made a significant modification to the intervention you are providing. For example from the provision of individual intensive therapy to a decision to review in 6 months; or if you have noted major change in the client, such as deterioration in performance; or if you decide to refer for other specialist opinion. A further reason for reporting would be in response to a request from another party, such as a lawyer, doctor, another professional or an education department.

The requirement for a report, whether initial, interim or closure, presents the clinician with a precious opportunity to bring together the evidence they have accrued about a client in a structured manner and to draw a comprehensive evaluation at a particular point in time. This is then written down in an appropriate form for the recipient of the report.

To guide the composition of the report it is helpful to ask a series of questions. The answers should inform the structure, length, content and distribution of the report that is sent.

## 1. What is the purpose of the report?

The report will differ depending on whether it is only informing or also requesting the recipient to do something, e.g. requesting additional information, opinion or referral to another agent. In cases where a request is being made, it should be supported with evidence to justify the request, such as the basis for the need for a hearing test, a psychological assessment, a teacher's report or medical opinion.

If the purpose is to transfer the case to a speech and language clinician in another authority, a very detailed report would be appropriate. Similarly, a report contributing to legal and provision decisions may include detail of specific assessments and treatments. Such elaboration would serve little usefulness to a recipient who requires a concise overview of the problems and functional effects of the disorder, the prognosis and proposals for future management, or basis for discharge.

## 2. What information should be included?

The report should only include what the recipient needs to know, and detail should be limited to that which is useful to them, and no more. The clinician must therefore be sensitive to the professional knowledge and to the current knowledge of the case that the recipient is likely to have. You can use technical terms without detailed explanations if you know that the other specialist has a common understanding with your own. The aim is to be concise. However, if knowledge base differs this must be accommodated by alternative expressions that will be understood. The purpose of reporting is not to confuse or appear pompous but to provide meaningful information. Where a variety of personnel are to receive the report the content, language and style will have to be appropriately modified.

Further, it is not necessary to include information that is already known to the recipient. Where you have sent an earlier report, do not repeat what has already been said. An initial reminder of a previous report ('Following my report dated...') can help the recipient locate the reference, but then all that is required of you is to indicate new information and changes that have occurred since the original report. Additionally, the recipient does not need to have information that they have documented or already shared with you repeated back to them.

### 3. Who should receive the report?

Initial reports must be sent to the referring agent. This may be a consultant, senior medical officer, GP, head teacher, a nursery manager, clinical psychologist or some other person. However, in the case of self-referral or carer referral the report is likely to be sent to the professional, perhaps the GP or head teacher, that the clinician considers would be particularly pertinent in the coordination of information affecting the client. Subsequent reports should also be sent to this person so that they are appropriately updated regarding speech and language support and the client.

Copies of reports can be sent to any agent if it is in the client's interest for that person to be cognisant of the information included. It is important to remember the wide network of professionals that should be kept informed. For example, for clients seen in hospital, a copy of the report to a consultant should be forwarded to the GP who is currently coordinating the care of the client outside hospital or will be after hospital discharge. In addition to reporting to a senior medical officer, copies should be sent to the school that is involved with a child's development on a day-to-day basis.

In some speech and language therapy services there may also be a requirement for a speech and language therapy manager to receive all reports. In this way there is a centralized access to information on clients and a valuable source of data for monitoring and audit.

It is essential at the end of the report to include a circulation list of all personnel who will be sent a copy. In this way each knows the extent to which others involved in the care of the client are being kept informed.

Finally, a copy of the report must always be kept on file in the client's case records.

### 4. What structure should the report follow?

Broadly, the report should include:

- An introduction, which includes client information (name, date of birth, address, hospital number), the detail of the primary recipient and a statement of the purpose of the report.
- A central part with subsections as necessary to cover a description of the communication problem, and past (if any) and present therapy.

- A summary of conclusions, including factors influencing prognosis and recommendations for future management.

Very commonly a service will have a standard form for reports. This uniformity helps other disciplines to become familiar with our ways. With standard forms headings and subheadings are likely to cover, for example, 'Background', 'Diagnosis', 'Receptive language', 'Expressive language', 'Treatment' and 'Summary and recommendations'. Where these headings do not best meet the needs of a particular case, another heading might be added. Even if a standard format is not common practice in a service, for example a letter format may be preferred, it is a still advisable to use headings.

### 5. What impression do we wish to convey?

The reputation of any service is influenced by the reports that are received by other personnel. This means that the report should be informative and also sensitive to the contributions of and demands on others. The style, form and content must not be in the vein of telling others what to do. Professional respect will be best achieved by a relevant, concise, well-organized and well-written report that acknowledges a need for working with others and welcomes an exchange of specialist knowledge and skills for the benefit of the client.

Short, clear sentences which progress in an orderly manner will help the reader assimilate information. Headings should be used to guide the reader through the content of the report, and an appropriate minimum of detail should be included within each section. Remember, it may only be the final summary paragraph that the reader considers is of interest or has time to look at. Make sure that this part of the report contains the key points you wish to make.

Finally, always check grammar and spelling. Not only are errors distracting to the reader, but also speech and language clinicians without a good command of written English will not attract respect from other disciplines.

## Information systems and statistics

Information systems include all the possible methods of recording, analysing and presenting data, whether manual or automated. In any business, there are three kinds of information that are important to guide planning and decision making. These are financial, manpower and activity, or productivity, data. Within health care, it is also necessary to collect clinical data. The wealth of data recorded in health information systems is capitalized on by countless agencies concerned with the health of the population and health care provision. For example:

- it is used to cost and evaluate services
- it contributes to epidemiology, that is the study of patterns of disorders, treatment and outcomes
- it is a source for research and audit related to health issues and health care practice
- it is applied in manpower planning and can help identify problems, for example in staffing levels and sickness
- it can reflect how local or government policies are being addressed.

Accurate, relevant and current data made available from all possible sources should increase the chance of appropriately based arguments for the management decisions that affect both health care employees and health care users.

Data collection by speech and language clinicians is essential to provide evidence of how the speech and language service resources are employed, and this information makes a major impact on service planning and endeavours to improve efficiency. Sometimes data are recorded manually on printed forms and submitted for central input into the computer system, and sometimes they are directly input into the system by the individual clinician. Variations depend on the sophistication of the information system of the particular authority. Although the methods, systems and codes used by different authorities vary, in essence the data related to clinicians and their day-to-day work will consist of two types of information, that associated with themselves and that associated with their clients.

Clinician information includes:

- identification details, such as a clinician code, personal information, appointment date and subsequent employment record
- daily client and non-client activities (e.g. face-to-face contact; telephone calls relating to clients; administration, from ordering stationery to completing statistics and report writing; liaison with other professionals; giving talks; attending staff meetings), the time spent on each activity and the location; holiday leave, study leave and sickness; and travel expenses.

Client information includes:

- identification details, such as name, date of birth, address, marital status, ethnic origin, language used, need for interpreter, referring agent, type of referral (new or rereferral), disorder category (e.g. language, fluency, voice, swallowing), education status.
- case management information, such as date of initial contact, nature (e.g. direct, indirect, individual, group) and length of subsequent contacts, and discharge details (e.g. mutual agreement between

clinician and client, failed to attend, refused treatment, death, loss of contact, assessment only, transferred out of the authority, treatment not available).

The primary purpose of coordinating information about clinicians and clients is to provide accurate, quantifiable centralized data about the service that is readily accessible to authorized personnel and agencies. From statistical analysis of the data on activity and caseloads, the features and costs of the speech and language service can be evaluated. In turn, this evidence can inform management decisions on quality improvements that are needed in provision, for example to support changes in patterns of referral or to increase efficiency to make best use of clinician time. The information is not only pertinent to the service itself, but will be used in making judgements about the distribution of resources across the authority. Thus it will be made available as appropriate to other interested parties, including the local authority and education departments. Additionally, to inform the national picture of health and related care provision it will be disseminated to the regional health department and the Department of Health.

In conclusion each speech and language clinician as an employee with a responsibility to an organization, as a professional with a responsibility to clients and as an individual concerned for fairness and effectiveness in the delivery of health care has a duty to be thorough in record keeping and reporting.

# Chapter 8
# Conclusions and
# Beginnings

The preceding chapters have laid the foundations of the professional practice of speech and language clinicians. Thought has been given to contexts of work; to relationships with clients, carers and other workers; to processes and practices of case and clinical management; and to issues of professional responsibility. With this background, and the vast amounts of theoretical and experiential learning that will be covered in the course of initial training, it is hoped the student speech and language clinician will gain the confidence, understanding and preparedness to enter employment as a speech and language clinician. But what next?

What does it mean to be a newly qualified speech and language clinician? It means that you have demonstrated that you have the appropriate knowledge, skills and attitudes to take responsibility for your own caseload and your own actions; to provide clients with a high quality of care; to work effectively with teams of speech and language clinicians and other workers; and to be an ambassador of your profession. It also means that you have a commitment to continuing your professional development. Your learning now begins.

### The transition from student clinician to clinician

No longer is there a supervising clinician who has ultimate responsibility for the decisions made and the actions taken on behalf of clients. No longer is there a carefully controlled caseload that a supervising clinician has selected to support your clinical development. No longer do you have time to conduct lengthy assessments and analyses on every aspect of communication of every client that is referred. No longer can you stand apart from the wide-ranging policies and procedures governing the organization in which your clinical work resides. No longer do you have a carefully organized curriculum of university- and practice-based learning managed by tutors and clinicians to guide your academic and professional development. Now it is your responsibility to use your time effectively so that you establish and maintain work networks, provide maximally effective care to maximum numbers of individuals with communication difficulties, reflect on your practice, and update your knowledge and skills to their potential. Frightening? No, exciting and challenging. With a calm, organized approach (even if the adrenaline runs riot) and the realization that your own resources and those provided by others are at your disposal, you can achieve what is expected of you. The following sections outline some of the support that should be available and, if they are not, the possibilities that should be negotiated with your manager in order to meet the recommendations of the professional body (RCSLT, 1996).

**Induction**

As a newly qualified member of staff  you should be taken carefully through information about the employing organization and the speech and language clinical service. You need to be briefed about:

- *Employment issues* You need to know what hours you are expected to work; your entitlement for annual leave and special leave for domestic, personal and family reasons; the procedures to follow in the event of sickness; the roles and responsibilities covered by your post; and how progression will be managed.
- *The management arrangements of the organization and the service* You need to know who you should contact according to the type of advice or agreements you are seeking, and to whom you are accountable and can look to for support. For example, who to contact with requests for leave, or for information about professional development opportunities, discussion of ideas you have regarding potential service delivery improvements, requests for engaging in research, advice on conflict at work and advice about specialist areas?
- *The policies and procedures operating in the organization and the service* You need to be familiar with the policy statement, that is the declaration of the purpose of the service and what it expects of staff in terms of professional responsibility. It is important that you are made aware of health and safety issues that affect you at work. For example, you need to know what to do in the event of exposure to challenging behaviour or infection; what hazards to be aware of and how they should be reported; how to protect confidentiality; and what guidance is in place to best ensure your personal safety. You also need to know about policies and procedures covering, for example, child protection, abuse of vulnerable adults, alcohol and drug use, equal opportunities, staff transport and allowances, ordering equipment, complaints and referral. Further, you need to be advised and trained in the data collection procedures that apply to the speech and language therapy service.

Commonly, you will be allowed some time to meet people, orient yourself to the locality in which you are working, review the caseload and gradually build up your workload. Often the demands from others and your own enthusiasm and concern to demonstrate your professional capabilities can lead to overload and stress and less effectiveness than desirable. An early lesson is to be realistic about what can be achieved; do not take on more than you can cope with. If you are uncertain what this might be, consult your line manager and establish what is appropriate and acceptable.

## Mentoring

Mentoring is generally put in place for newly qualified staff, and also for those returning to work after a career break and for staff taking on a new specialist role. It can operate in various ways. In general a mentor is a more senior colleague, but not the line manager. Mentoring can take place through meetings with peers as well as the mentor. It aims to enable the individual to work through concerns, clarify understanding of policies and procedures, question and reflect on practice, learn from others, and have her development monitored, and so progress towards fuller clinical autonomy.

## Rotation, shadowing, working with peers and other workplace learning

More than anywhere else, professional development occurs within the daily work of the clinician. Every day the clinician will reflect on what she does, formulate hypotheses about how to improve practice, and try out and evaluate different ways of working. Practice does not make perfect, it provides opportunities to continually reflect and change. A clinician should constantly seek new learning and ways to develop. A good clinician is a questioning clinician.

In some services there are arrangements for new staff to be employed on a rotational basis. Thus, a clinician might work for four months in a health clinic setting, four months in a hospital setting and four months in a school or nursery setting. This provides opportunities to build on the grounding of clinical experience of a variety of client groups gained as an undergraduate, but with the authority and freedom in decision making of a qualified member of staff. It also allows the new clinician to become familiar with personnel, facilities and practices across the service and gives time to define work and career preferences. It will provide a foundation for negotiations with the manger to establish how service needs and the personal and professional aspirations of the clinician can best be met.

As a student clinician you will have found it extremely valuable to shadow and observe how experienced clinicians spend their time and how they relate to clients and other people within the scope of their work. In this context you can learn so much without having to take responsibility for the activities involved. As a new clinician, or when learning a new specialism, shadowing can once again provide a very welcome and rich opportunity for learning. Shadowing not only requires carefully structured observation, but also time to discuss and reflect on what was observed. Also it should involve time in researching the literature on related theory and practice. The library does not get left behind once the word 'qualified' is attached to you.

Throughout your career, shadowing more experienced clinicians, those who practise different approaches to yourself, or those with specialist expertise that you have not developed is an excellent way to learn. Some speech and language clinical services with a highly specialist department (e.g. in cleft palate, dysphagia or voice disorder) may take this even further. They may offer opportunities for staff from other authorities to spend time in shadowing and other activity in a training programme with a view to developing similar specialist services on returning to their home authority. Obviously while you are away there are costs to your own organization for such development opportunities. However, the absence of one clinician can provide an opening for another person to experience a new area of work if they take on the vacant position on a temporary basis. We all become stale if we remain in the same role too long. Even a short break can refresh the clinician, and variety will bring different experiences that can stimulate reflection and change, whether moving on or back to post.

Another invaluable opportunity for learning with and from others is by working alongside another speech and language clinician, for example running a group. From the model of the techniques, ideas and behaviours applied by the other professional, particularly if followed up by discussion, you can see new and different ways of working, reflect on your current practices and modify your approach to the advantage of clients. Clinicians must be constantly open to improvement and change .

**Time management training**

Clinical work requires balancing a range of demands and responsibilities and the tight deadlines that accompany them. As a new clinician it can be daunting to decide just how long you can spend on a particular activity, and which activities and which people have to wait or not be involved in your scheme of work. With experience you will learn how long aspects of your work take, you will learn to do things more quickly, you will do things more efficiently and you will not get so stressed if things get left undone if you are confident that your priorities were correct. There will never be sufficient resources to do everything that you wish to do. Your educational background probably taught you the ideals of how to be thorough, but in practice thoroughness has to be weighed against the demands of waiting lists, throughput, attendance at meetings, giving talks, a commitment to administration, and your personal and professional development. Time constraints mean that only that which is essential can be done. Sometimes you will not be able to do what would be interesting, that extra in-depth assessment or long counselling session, if it means other clients have to be neglected. Most experienced clinicians have a personal strategy of time management. It may be helpful early in your initial employment to work through issues of time management with a mentor or peers, or to negotiate specific staff development, perhaps an in-service training course, in this field.

### Clinical supervision (non-managerial supervision)

The aim of clinical supervision is to maximize clinical effectiveness through reflective practice. While mentoring enables the new clinician, returner or new specialist to reflect and learn and be guided through a particular stage of professional development, clinical supervision is applicable outside of such stages. It can be relevant throughout the career of the professional. Depending on the resources allocated to the practice by the employing organization, clinical supervision may be incorporated within the workload of every member of staff, or opportunities may be made available for staff to receive clinical supervision on a voluntary basis. In some organisations it may not be possible to access clinical supervision.

The practice involves pairing a clinician with a supervisor who has had training in the required techniques. These parties will negotiate a contract, that is the ground rules for the supervision. This may cover the timing and duration, place, type, method of recording, skills and techniques, confidentiality, structure of sessions and emergency strategies (e.g. whether contact outside of agreed sessions is acceptable). Clinical supervision should not be confused with counselling, although some of the techniques used by counsellors, such as listening, exploration and reflection, may be used in interactions between the supervisor and the person being supervised. Clinical supervision is distinct from the relationship with a manager. It does not involve directing or monitoring the work of the clinician. Instead it is a forum of open discussion, based on trust and confidentiality, which provides professional support. It enables the clinician to focus on work-related difficulties, challenge coping strategies, reflect on practice and explore ways to improve service delivery. It can help clinicians to use resources more successfully, manage workloads more effectively and improve practice, and it can reduce the chances of burn out. Clinical supervision thus contributes to the process of continual learning and personal and professional development.

### Managerial supervision

Every speech and language clinician will have a manager to whom they are accountable. The manager will provide guidance and direction, and will monitor the clinician's work. This person will have a concern for the needs of the service and clients, as well as the needs of individual members of staff. Guidance, negotiation and decisions about work patterns and policies and procedures will be channelled through this manager. The manager will have a key role in facilitating your personal and professional development and ensuring you make the best possible contribution to the service. The relationship should be supportive and conducted through both informal and formal contacts. As well as ongoing discussions about your progress and development, formal meetings will be set out to review your development. These meetings vary in name and form within different services, e.g. individual performance review, staff development review or appraisal.

### Individual performance review (IPR), staff development review, appraisal

The meetings to review your development as a member of staff are an opportunity to:

* review your job description
* review what you have achieved since the last meeting and consider how far you have met previously agreed objectives
* review any difficulties you have experienced in carrying out your duties
* identify training and development that would support you
* discuss your aspirations and career expectations
* clarify with your manager what the service requires of you
* agree objectives and the timescale within which they should be achieved.

### Continuing personal and professional development

Responsible professionals will be highly motivated to engage in a wide range of learning opportunities in order to develop practice and improve service delivery. Reflective practice, that is the constant review of one's practice and the seeking of learning opportunities to increase knowledge, refine present skills and acquire new skills, and to apply these in the workplace, is vital for effective practice. We have already mentioned a variety of contexts for personal and professional development – induction, mentoring, work rotation, shadowing, peer discussion, peer working, workplace experience and training, non-managerial supervision, managerial supervision, reading and in-service training. Course and conference attendance, research activity, and interest and audit group involvement are among the many activities that can contribute to personal and professional development. Many of these activities can shape continuing professional development for the clinician.

Continuing professional development is the process whereby the clinician defines the professional development goals that are necessary not only to remain competent to practise, but to grow in competence and offer a greater level and scope of expertise. The goals will normally be guided by the agreements made with the manager within the staff review process. For example, for a particular year in the career of a clinician working with a paediatric caseload in health clinics and nurseries, goals might be set as follows:

- to update knowledge and skills in working with children with language disorders
- to advance knowledge of policy issues affecting the care of children
- to develop expertise in working with others
- to improve report writing
- to develop ways for improving the integration of family members in therapy.

The clinician must then ensure that she identifies and engages in activities that will assist the attainment of the stated goals. For example the above clinician might achieve the goal 'to improve report writing' by the following activities:

- attendance at an in-service course on report writing
- involvement in an audit meeting to identify good practice in report writing
- reading reports of more experienced colleagues
- discussing own reports with a manager.

The Royal College of Speech and Language Therapists (RCSLT) states that a full-time speech and language clinician must devote the equivalent of 10 (half-day) sessions per year on relevant continuing personal and professional development activity (RCSLT, 1996). Once you realize how much development is achieved within your day-to-day work and does not depend on course or conference attendance or formal research, it is easy to establish a profile of continuing professional development that far exceeds the minimum stated requirement for professional registration. A range of possible activities are identified below.

*Courses, workshops, seminars and conferences*

A course could require anything from working towards a postgraduate degree to undertaking a non-certificated, that is non-assessed, course that may be only a few hours in duration. Courses may involve learning with non-speech and language clinicians. They may be offered through a variety of contexts, such as lectures, workshops or seminars, and in some instances through distance learning. They may be conducted as an in-service provision in your own organization, or delivered by some other organization, such as another health provider, a private company or a university.

When a series of sessions is offered intensively, generally on a large scale, the term conference will apply. Like many forms of courses, these offer excellent opportunities not only to learn from arranged sessions of presentations and seminars, but also from informal contacts between sessions and, particularly in residential settings, the exchanges that take place at the end of the day. It is during the informal meetings that networks can be built that will support your work. Conferences, and many courses, commonly provide opportunities for suppliers to display books, assessments, therapy materials and information leaflets relevant to the specialist area(s) covered, and hence are a valuable source of updating.

### Books, journals and articles

Reading about aspects of professional practice is an obvious way to update knowledge. You should regularly read professional and specialist journals, research into specific theories and approaches when you need more knowledge to manage an individual case, and make time to discover and read books that will inform your professional practice. It is also important to remember that learning from reading can be enriched by discussion, and that if you share what you have read with others it will both help to clarify your understanding and contribute to a greater understanding across a group of colleagues. Journal clubs are sometimes developed for this purpose, quite often as an informal network, and may perhaps be held during lunchtimes. The 'club' might be restricted to speech and language clinicians, but more commonly will extend to other personnel in the workplace. Members take turns to talk about interesting research papers as a starting point for group discussion. This means you are exposed to ideas and practices that you may not have otherwise focused on that may stimulate new approaches in your own work.

It is often from the combination of an enquiring mind, clinical experience and the opportunity to read and discuss with other colleagues that the seeds are sown for active research .

### Research

The possibility that you will become involved in formal research at some time or other in your career is today greater than ever. The value of a scientific investigation of theory and practice is now well recognized both for informing professional practice and for the personal and professional development of practitioners. There are as many things to research as there are problems generated by the people for whom you have responsibility as a speech and language clinician. Thus you may be disappointed that your research contribution seems to make such a small impact when compared to all the questions that remain unanswered. Remember that you are at least making a contribution, and that the experience of research will itself shape your own thinking, knowledge and understanding.

Research might be conducted as an individual or in collaboration with others from your own or other disciplines. It might be undertaken with a view to gaining a research degree. You might engage in funded research, perhaps supported by monies from the research and development funds of your organization or the region, or from national research award bodies. You might conduct either large- or small-scale research with the intention of presenting the work at a meeting, seminar or conference, or publishing it in a paper that will be read by fellow speech and language clinicians or other people for whom the study has relevance.

McConkey (1991: 4–5) suggests that within speech and language clinical practice there are three main areas of research:

1. Client characteristics, such as:
   - descriptions of language characteristics
   - relationships of certain language patterns to certain disorder categories
   - surveys, for example of geographical distributions of certain disorders.
2. Effectiveness of what we do, such as:
   - pre- and post-therapy comparisons
   - comparisons of different types of therapy
   - the nature of the therapy that brought about change.
3. Service effectiveness, such as:
   - consideration of different intensities of input
   - the use of different personnel to offer input.

We have stressed throughout this text that, as a speech and language clinician, your work with clients will be informed by a scientific approach. Every time you see a client and go through the scientific process of investigating the nature of that client's problems, recording what you are doing and planning therapy based on what you discover, you are 'doing research'. The difference between this and the more formalized procedure of research is based mainly on, first, the systematic nature of the process and, second, the dissemination of the information.

The systematic nature of the process includes:

- thorough exploration and a literature search to establish a problem to be investigated, questions to be answered and/or a hypothesis to be tested
- conducting carefully designed subject selection and data collection procedures
- presenting and analysing the results
- drawing conclusions from the findings that will contribute to understandings and identify ways forward for the progression of related research.

The traditional philosophy behind scientific enquiry, or research, is that of positivism, the fact that knowledge can only be derived from empirical, that is observable, evidence. For example, establishing the causes of a disorder from examination of case data, establishing the features of a disorder from an analysis of a speech sample, establishing how people change as an outcome of intervention from testing performance. This framework informs a great deal of the research carried out by speech and language clinicians. Additionally, there is a wealth of understanding that cannot be observed and measured that is equally significant in the development of professional issues and practice. For example, we not only want to know about change due to intervention from quantitative measures of the test results or observed performance of clients, but we also need to consider their opinion about the process they were taken through. Thus qualitative research which investigates the opinions, attitudes, perceptions and beliefs of subjects plays a vital role in the development of professional practice.

## The dissemination of the information

We fail in our responsibility as a researcher and as a professional if the outcomes of the investigation are not shared with, or disseminated to, other people. Researching is not only about striving for personal development, but also striving to make a contribution to our own profession and beyond and to future research.

There are many ways of sharing your work with others; the choice will be guided by the size, type and purpose of the study and the range of people that you hope to reach. Written dissemination might be in the form of a research report or dissertation of a research degree; an article in the newsletter published by specific groups of professionals or agencies that you wish to influence; a poster at a conference; or a paper in a journal. Alternatively, dissemination might be achieved through oral presentation, such as at a seminar, conference, workshop, discussion group or meeting. It is important to remember that research will not only require a commitment from you, but also an investment in you by your employer. This will only have been granted if the research is perceived to be of value to both parties. You have a duty to recognize that investment by making public the outcome of that investment.

Whatever sort of researcher you turn out to be, it is worth reflecting on the list of qualities summarized by McConkey (1991):

- The researcher is a questioning person, not contented with the status quo.
- The researcher is creative and enjoys thinking of new approaches.
- The person who researches is a risk taker, prepared to discover uncomfortable truths.

- Because much of research is about being organized, the researcher is a good manager.
- The researcher must be diplomatic and able to negotiate with a wide range of people.
- The researcher must be numerate and happy to deal with numbers and figures.
- Finally, the researcher is a plodder, willing to just keep going until the project has been completed.

You may not recognize all of these qualities in yourself, but you will be able to relate to some of them, and others with whom you work will probably relate to different ones. This is why research, or at least some aspects of the process, is best carried out with others, and why you should always seek support, whether from a research supervisor, research coordinator, experienced researchers and statisticians, or colleagues.

### Special interest groups (SIGs), local groups and audit

The benefits of learning with and from others cannot be overemphasized. To this end there are several types of formally arranged networks or groups that you may be able or even required to access. Special interest groups consist of clinicians who have a common specialist interest. They may be for clinicians working in special schools or in mainstream schools; clinicians working with adults with learning disability, cleft palate, head and neck disorders, semantic-pragmatic disorders or dysphagia; or clinicians with an interest in approaches such as cognitive neuropsychology. SIGs are generally organized by teams of interested clinicians in a region. However, some are organized at a national level. Meetings may involve guest speakers and discussion, as well as proactive activities such as the development of information leaflets. Very often it is difficult to decide which group to join when several relate to the range of your clinical interests. Remember that involvement in groups such as this demands time, often beyond attendance at meetings, if you are going to benefit and contribute maximally. First, beware of over-commitment. Second, take a responsible attitude to the use of your time. Professional development activity must be agreed with your manager.

Local groups are formed by clinicians in a local region. The members will have a range of interests, but their common objective will be to share experiences and practices and to promote the profession. Projects such as those that raise awareness about communication disability are often taken on by these groups. Like SIGs, the presentations arranged are often open to any interested clinician and not confined to those in the locality or with membership of the group.

In addition to the individual clinician striving for the greatest effectiveness within her own case management, audit groups are commonly set up within speech and language clinical services to enable clinicians from a defined discipline, or from across a service, to jointly evaluate or audit the outcomes of clinical activity and the structure and processes of the service. Multidisciplinary audit groups may look at the overall care of clients from one particular disorder category, for example stroke. In this way best practice can be identified and change proposed and implemented following a peer group exercise. At the same time, it is an opportunity for the individual clinician to learn about the practices and experiences of others and to explore alternatives, which in turn contributes to personal and professional development. It will be helpful at this point to explain a little further about audit.

> Clinical audit is a process in which doctors, nurses and other health professionals systematically review, and where necessary make changes to, the care and treatment they provide to patients (Audit Office, 1995).

Audit enables professionals to evaluate whether the standards set for the service that they are delivering are being met. They will consider the quality of the service provided in terms of its:

- *Effectiveness*, whether the service is achieving its objectives, for example providing treatment that benefits the clients.
- *Efficiency*, whether the service is cost effective, for example maximizing the numbers of clients seen and the range of services provided within the budget.
- *Equity*, whether the service is fairly provided, for example across geographical, social or ethnic groups.
- *Appropriateness*, whether the service is relevant to the needs of the community it serves.
- *Acceptability*, whether the activities of the service are acceptable to groups and society at large.
- *Accessibility*, whether the service is offered at times and locations that suit the community it serves.

Audit can be carried out in many different ways. Random sampling of reports to referring agents or of speech and language case records; surveys of accommodation, equipment and client satisfaction; staff appraisal or individual performance review; peer observation, case discussion and information sharing about clinical approaches and problems are among the many means by which audit can be conducted. An essential aspect of audit is that findings are recorded and evaluated and reported to managers, together with recommendations, so that action can be taken to improve service delivery. A useful manual that guides clinicians who may be new to the process of audit has been published by the College of Speech and Language Therapists (1993).

Audit is yet another activity that provides the clinician with opportunities to learn, reflect and achieve personal and professional development, and at the same time contribute to the delivery of a quality service.

## Conclusion

This text can only provide a taster of speech and language clinical practice. As a professional you have extensive responsibility – to your clients, to your employer, to yourself and to your colleagues. At times it will be daunting, at times stressful, but for the most part clinicians discover that the challenges and rewards far outweigh the anxieties. At the same time you will realize from this chapter that informal and formal support systems are always on hand, not least those provided by the network of speech and language clinicians and other personnel in your working life. This support and your own professional attitude, commitment to team working, natural empathy, individual personality and all the knowledge and skills you continually develop, will keep you on course.

This book has attempted to provide a framework for your working practices, your interventions with clients, and your personal and professional development. Armed with this information you should be able to launch yourself with confidence into clinical work.

# References

Alcorn M, Harratt T, Martin W, Dodd B (1995) Intensive group therapy: efficacy of a whole-language approach. In Dodd B, Differential Diagnosis and Treatment of Children with Speech Disorders. London: Whurr.

Allen C (1992) In their own times... Nursery World.4 June, 12–13.

Ambrose N, Yairi E, Cox N (1993) Genetic aspects of early childhood stuttering. Journal of Speech and Hearing Research 36: 701–6.

American Speech-Language-Hearing Association and the International Association of Logopedics and Phoniatrics (1994) An International Directory of Education for Speech-Language Pathologists (Speech Therapists/Logopedists/Orthophonites). Maryland: ASHA.

Audit Office (1995) Press Notice 64/950 on NHS (England): Clinical Audit in England.

Bannister D (1982) Knowledge of self. In Purser H (ed.), Psychology for Speech Therapists. London: British Psychological Society.

Barker P (1996) Basic Family Therapy, 3rd edn. London: Collins.

Barry C (1991) Acquired disorders of reading and spelling: a cognitive neuropsychological perspective. In Code C (ed.), The Characteristics of Aphasia. Hove, East Sussex: Lawrence Erlbaum.

Beech J, Harding L, Hilton-Jones D (eds) (1993) Assessment in Speech and Language Therapy. London: Routledge.

Belbin M (1993) Team Roles at Work. Oxford: Butterworth Heinemann.

Bishop DVM (1989) Test for the Reception of Grammar, 2nd edn (1st edn 1983). Manchester: Department of Psychology, University of Manchester.

Bower T (1987) Special Educational Needs and Resource Management. London: Croom Helm.

Breakwell G (1990) Interviewing. London: Routledge, BPS Books.

Brechin A, Swain J (1988) Professional/client relationships: creating a working alliance with people with learning disabilities. Disability, Handicap and Society 3: 213–26.

Byers Brown B, Edwards M (1989) Developmental Language Disorders. London: Whurr.

Byers Brown B, Gilbert J (1989) The profession at work. In Leahy M (ed.), Disorders of Communication: the Science of Intervention. London: Taylor and Francis.

Byng S (1995) What is aphasia therapy? In Code C, Muller D, Treatment of Aphasia: From Theory to Practice. London: Whurr.

Byng S, Black M (1995) What makes a therapy? Some parameters of therapeutic intervention in aphasia. European Journal of Disorders of Communication 30: 303–16.

Care Sector Consortium (1996) Consultation Document: Development of National Occupational Standards for Three Groups of Health Care Practitioners.

Carlomagno S (1994) Pragmatic Approaches to Aphasia Therapy. London: Whurr.

College of Speech and Language Therapists (1991) Communicating Quality: Professional Standards for Speech and Language Therapists. London: College of Speech and Language Therapists.

College of Speech and Language Therapists (1993) Audit: A Manual for Speech and Language Therapists. London: College of Speech and Language Therapists.

Connard P (1984) P.A.I.P. The Preverbal Assessment-Intervention Profile. Austin, Texas: pro-ed.

Cooper EB, Cooper CS (1985) Personalized Fluency Control Therapy. Leicester: (Developmental Learning Materials) Taskmaster.

Cooper J, Moodley M, Reynell J (1978) Helping Language Development. London: Edward Arnold.

Costello J (1993) Behavioural Treatment of Stuttering Children. In Curlee R (ed.) Stuttering and Related Disorders of Fluency. New York: Thieme Medical.

Council of Local Education Authorities (1994) Letter to Jeffrey, DFE, 10 February. London: CLEA.

Crystal D (1982) Profiling Linguistic Disability. London: Edward Arnold.

Crystal D, Fletcher P, Garman M (1989) Grammatical Analysis of Language Disability, 2nd edn. London: Whurr.

Crystal D, Varley R (1993) Introduction to Language Pathology, 3rd edn. London: Whurr.

Dalton P (1994) Counselling People with Communication Problems. London: Sage.

Dalton P, Dunnett G (1992) A Psychology for Living: Personal Construct Theory for Professionals and Clients. Chichester: John Wiley and Sons.

Davies P, van der Gaag A (1992) The professional competence of speech therapists: III skills and skill mix possibilities. Clinical Rehabilitation 6: 311–24.

Davis GA, Wilcox MJ (1981) Incorporating parameters of natural conversation in aphasia treatment. In Chapey R (ed.), Language Intervention Strategies in Adult Aphasia. Baltimore: Williams & Wilkins.

Davis GA. Wilcox MJ (1985) Adult Aphasia Rehabilitation: Applied Pragmatics. Windsor: NFER-Nelson.

Dawkins R (1986) The Blind Watchmaker. London: Penguin.

de Bono E (1985) Tactics: The Art and Science of Success. London: Collins.

Dean EC, Howell J (1986) Developing linguistic awareness: a theoretically based approach to phonological disorders. British Journal of Disorders of Communication 21: 223–38.

Dean EC, Howell J, Waters D, Reid J (1995) Metaphon: a metalinguistic approach to the treatment of phonological disorder in children. Clinical Linguistics and Phonetics 9: 283–321.

Department of Education and Science (1981) Education Act. London: HMSO.

Department of Education (1994) Code of Practice on the Identification and Assessment of Special Educational Needs. London: Department for Education.

Department of Health (1993) Mental Illness: Key Area Handbook. London: DoH.

Dockerill J, Henry C (1993) Assessment of mentally handicapped individuals In Beech J, Harding L, Hilton-Jones D (eds), Assessment in Speech and Language Therapy. London: Routledge.

Dodd B (1995) Procedures for classification of subgroups of speech disorder. In Dodd B, Differential Diagnosis and Treatment of Children with Speech Disorder. London: Whurr.

Dryden W (1990) Individual Therapy: A Handbook. Milton Keynes: Open University Press.

Duncan D (ed.) (1989) Working with Bilingual Language Disability. London: Chapman and Hall.

Dunn LM, Dunn LM, Whetton C, Pintile D (1982) British Picture Vocabulary Scale. Windsor: NFER-Nelson.

Edwards JA (1993) Principles and contrasting systems of discourse transcription. In Edwards JA, Lampert MD (eds), Talking Data: Transcription and Coding in Discourse Research. Hillsdale, NJ: Lawrence Erlbaum.

Edwards S, Fletcher P, Garman M, Hughes A, Letts C, Sinka I (1997) The Reynell Developmental Language Scales III. Windsor: NFER-Nelson.

Egan G (1978) The Skilled Helper: A Systematic Approach to Skilled Helping. California: Brooks Cole.

Egan G (1994) The Skilled Helper: A Problem-management Approach to Helping, 5th edn. California: Brooks Cole.

Enderby P (1992) Outcome measures in speech therapy: impairment, disability, handicap and distress. Health Trends 24(2): 61–6.

Enderby P, Emerson J (1995) Does Speech and Language Therapy Work? A Review of the Literature. London: Whurr.

Enderby P, John A (1997) Therapy Outcome Measures (Speech and Language Therapy). London: Singular Press.

Fabb N (1994) Sentence Structure. London: Routledge.

Fawcus M (ed.) (1992) Group Encounters in Speech and Language Therapy. Kibworth: Far Communications.

Fielder M (1993) FIRST Screening Test. Abergavenny: Nevill Hall Hospital.

Finkelstein V (1993) From curing or caring to defining disabled people. In Walmsley J, Reynolds J, Shakespeare P, Woolfe R (eds) Health, Welfare and Practice: Reflecting on Roles and Relationships. London: Sage/Open University.

Foxen T, McBrien J (1981) Training Staff in Behavioural Methods. Trainee Workbook. Manchester: Manchester University Press.

Fransella F, Dalton P (1990) Personal Construct Counselling in Action. London: Sage.

Frederickson N, Frith U, Reason R (1997) Phonological Assessment Battery. Windsor: NFER-Nelson.

Gardner H (1997) Are your minimal pairs too neat? The dangers of phonemicisation in phonology therapy. European Journal of Disorders of Communication 32: 167–75.

Geekie P, Raban B (1994) Language learning at home and school. In Galloway C, Richards B, Input and Interaction in Language Acquisition. Cambridge: Cambridge University Press.

Gibbard D (1994) Parental-based intervention with pre-school language delayed children. European Journal of Disorders of Communication 29(2): 131–50.

Gipps C, Gross H, Goldstein H (1987) Warnock's Eighteen Per Cent. London: The Falmer Press.

Girolametto L (1988) Developing dialogue skills: the effects of a conversational model of language intervention. In Marfo K (ed.) Parent-Child Interaction and Developmental Disabilities. New York: Praeger.

Gorrie B, Parkinson E (1995) Phonological Awareness Procedure. Ponteland, Northumberland: STASS Publications.

Green R (1992) Supervision as an essential part of practice. Human Communication February, 21–2.

Gregory H (1979) Controversies about Stuttering Therapy. Baltimore: University Park Press.

Grunwell P (1985) Phonological Assessment of Child Speech (PACS). Windsor: NFER-Nelson.

Grunwell P (1987) Clinical Phonology, 2nd edn. London: Croom Helm.

Hall DMB (1989) Health for All Children: A Programme for Child Surveillance. Oxford: Open University Press.

Hargie O, Saunders C, Dickson D. (1994) Social Skills in Interpersonal Communication, 3rd edn. London: Routledge.

Harley T (1995) The Psychology of Language: From Data to Theory. London: Taylor and Francis.

Harrow J, Shaw M (1992) The manager faces the consumer. In Willcocks L, Harrow J (eds), Rediscovering Public Services Management. London: McGraw-Hill.

Hawkins P, Shohet R (1992) Supervision in the Helping Professions. Buckingham: Open University Press.

Heron J (1990) Helping the Client: A Creative Practical Guide. London: Sage.

Houghton D, McColgan M (1995) Working with Children. London: Collins Educational.

Howard D, Hatfield F (1987) Aphasia Therapy: Historical and Contemporary Issues. Hove and London: Lawrence Erlbaum.

Howell J, Dean E (1994) Treating Phonological Disorders in Children: Metaphon – Theory to Practice, 2nd edn. London: Whurr.

Hubbell RD (1981) Children's Language Disorders: An Integrated Approach. Engelwood Cliffs, NJ: Prentice-Hall.

Huczynski AA, Buchanan DA (1993) Organizational Behaviour: An Introductory Text, 2nd edn. London: Prentice-Hall.

Hudson B (1987) Collaboration in social welfare: a framework for analysis. Policy and Practice 15: 175–82.

Huntington J (1981) Social Work and General Medical Practice. London: Allen and Unwin.

Ingham R (1984) Stuttering and Behavior Therapy: Current Status and Experimental Foundations. San Diego: College-Hill Press.

Ingram D (1989) Phonological Disability in Children, 2nd edn. London: Whurr.

Institute of Medicine (1996) Primary Care: America's Health in a New Era. IOM Report.

Jacques D (1991) Learning in Groups. London/New York: Kegan Paul.

Jeffree D (1996) Observation of play in the early assessment and development of children with severe learning difficulties. In Fawcus M (ed.), Children with Learning Difficulties: A Collaborative Approach to their Education and Management. London: Whurr.

Johnson D, Johnson F (1991) Joining Together: Group Theory and Group Skills, 4th edn. Englewood Cliffs, NJ: Prentice-Hall.

Jowett S, Evans C (1996) Speech and Language Therapy Services for Children. Windsor: NFER-Nelson.

Kelly G (1963) A Theory of Personality: The Psychology of Personal Constructs. New York: Norton.

Kelly J, Local J (1989) Doing Phonology. Manchester: Manchester University Press.

Keresz A (1982) The Western Aphasia Battery (WAB). New York: Grune and Stratton.

Kineen L (1994) A journey towards a quality service. Journal of Clinical Speech and Language Studies 4(1): 45–55.

Knowles W, Masidlover M (1982) The Derbyshire Language Scheme. Education Office, Ripley, Derbyshire.

Ladefoged P (1982) A Course in Phonetics, 2nd edn. San Diego: Harcourt Brace Jovanovich.

Lahey M (1988) Language Disorders and Language Development. New York: Macmillan.

Lawson R, Pring T, Fawcus M (1993) The effects of short courses in modifying attitudes of adult and adolescent stutterers to communication. European Journal of Disorders of Communication 28(3): 299–308.

Leahy M (1989) The philosophy of intervention. In Leahy M (ed.), Disorders of Communication: the Science of Intervention. London: Taylor and Francis.

Leahy M (1995) Self-perception: the therapist in the process of change. In Wirz S (ed.), Perceptual Approaches to Communication Disorders. London: Whurr.

Lees J, Urwin S (1997) Children with Language Disorders, 2nd edn. London: Whurr.

Lesser R (1992) The making of logopedists: an international survey. Folia Phoniatrica 44: 105–25.

Levelt W (1989) Speaking: From Intention to Articulation. Cambridge, MA: MIT Press.

Lubinski R (1994) Environmental systems approach to adult aphasia. In Chapey R (ed.), Language Intervention Strategies in Adult Aphasia, 3rd edn. Baltimore/London: Williams & Wilkins.

McConkey R (1991) Practitioners as researchers. Journal of Clinical Speech and Language Studies 1: 1–15.

McDaniel D, McKee C, Smith Cairns H (1996) Methods for Assessing Children's Syntax. Cambridge, MA: MIT Press.

Marschark M, Siple P, Lillo-Martin D, Campbell R, Everhart V (1997) Relations of Language and Thought: The View from Sign Language and Deaf Children. Oxford: Oxford University Press.

Martin S (1987) Working with Dysphonics. Oxon: Winslow Press.

Miller J (1981) Assessing Language Production in Children. Baltimore: University Park Press.

Miller N, Docherty G (1995) Acquired neurogenic speech disorders: applying linguistics to treatment. In Grundy K (ed.), Linguistics in Clinical Practice, 2nd edn. London: Whurr.

Onslow M (1992) Identification of early stuttering: issues and suggested strategies. American Journal of Speech and Language Pathology 1: 21–7.

Parasuraman A, Zeithaml V, Berry L (1985) A conceptual model of service quality and its implications for future research. Journal of Marketing 19(6); 5–11.

Parker A, Irlam S (1995) Speech intelligibility and deafness: the skills of listener and speaker. In Wirz S (ed.), Perceptual Approaches to Communication Disorders. London: Whurr.

Pennington L, Windett W (1994) Outcomes of 'My turn to speak – a team approach to AAC'. RCSLT Bulletin 503: 12–14.

Perkins M, Howard S (1995) Case Studies in Clinical Linguistics. London: Whurr.

Phelps-Terasaki D, Phelps-Gunn T (1992) Test of Pragmatic Language. Austin, Texas: pro-ed.

Pinker S (1994) The Language Instinct. London: Penguin.

Priestley P, McGuire J (1983) Learning to Help: Basic Skills Exercises. London: Tavistock Publications.

Prochaska J, DiClemente C (1986) Towards a comprehensive model of change. In Miller W, Heather N (eds), Treating Addictive Behaviours. New York: Plenum Press.

Rogers CR (1951) Client-centered Therapy. London: Constable.

Rossiter D (1997) Global outcome measures, global warning. RCSLT Bulletin 543: 8–9.

Roulstone S (1988) The speech therapist. In Coupe J, Porter J (eds), The Education of Children with Severe Learning Difficulties. London: Croom Helm.

Royal College of Speech and Language Therapists (1996) Communicating Quality 2: Professional Standards for Speech and Language Therapists. London: RCSLT.

Rustin L, Cook F, Spence R (1995) The Management of Stuttering in Adolescence: A Communication Skills Approach. London: Whurr.

Sarno MT (1969) The Functional Communication Profile. New York University Medical Centre.

Sears DO, Peplau A, Freedman JL, Taylor SE (1988) Social Psychology, 6th edn. Englewood Cliffs, NJ: Prentice-Hall.

Selekman M (1993) Pathways to Change: Brief Therapy Solutions with Difficult Adolescents. New York/London: The Guilford Press.

Semel E, Wiig E, Secord W (1987) Clinical Evaluation of Language Fundamentals, revised edn. The Psychological Corporation, San Antonio: Harcourt Brace Jovanovich.

Sheehan JG (1975) Conflict theory and avoidance reduction therapy. In Eisenson J (ed.), Stuttering: A Second Symposium. New York: Harper and Row.

Shriberg L, Lof G (1991) Reliability studies in broad and narrow phonetic transcription. Clinical Linguistics and Phonetics 5: 225–79.

Snowling M, Stackhouse J (eds) (1996) Dyslexia, Speech and Language: A Practitioner's Handbook. London: Whurr.

Square-Storer P (ed.) (1989) Acquired Apraxia of Speech on Adults. London: Taylor and Francis.

Stackhouse J, Wells B (1997) Children's Speech and Literacy Problems: A psycholinguistic framework. London: Whurr.

Stengelhofen J (1993) Teaching Students in Clinical Settings. London: Chapman and Hall.

Street E (1994) Counselling for Family Problems. London: Sage.

Tuckman BW (1965) Developmental sequences in small groups. Psychological Bulletin 63: 384–99.

Van der Gaag A, Davies P (1992a) The professional competence of speech therapists: II knowledge base. Clinical Rehabilitation 6: 215–24.

Van der Gaag A, Davies, P (1992b) The professional competence of speech therapists: IV attitude and attribute base. Clinical Rehabilitation 6: 325–31.

Van Riper C (1973) The Treatment of Stuttering. Engelwood Cliffs, NJ: Prentice-Hall.

Van Riper C, Emerick L (1984) Speech Correction: An Introduction to Speech Pathology and Audiology, 5th edn. Engelwood Cliffs, NJ: Prentice-Hall.

Vogel D, Carter J (1995) The Effects of Drugs on Communication Disorders. San Diego: Singular Press.

Wall M, Myers F (1984) Clinical Management of Childhood Stuttering. Baltimore: University Park Press.

Ward S (1994) The validation of a treatment method for language delay in infants under one year of age. Paper presented at CPLOL Conference, Antwerp.

Warnock Report: DES. Committee of Inquiry into the Education of Handicapped Children and Young People (1978) Special Educational Needs. London: HMSO.

Wertz RT, La Pointe L, Rosenbek JC (1984) Apraxia of Speech in Adults: The Disorder and Its Management. San Diego: Singular Press.

Whitaker DS (1989) Using Groups to Help People. London: Routledge.

White M, East K (1983) The Wessex Revised Portage Language Checklist. Windsor: NFER-Nelson.

Whitworth A, Perkins L, Lesser R (1997) Conversation Analysis Profile for People with Aphasia. London: Whurr.

Williams J (1993) What is a profession: experience versus expertise. In Walmsley J, Shakespeare T, Woolfe R (eds) Health, Welfare and Practice. London: Sage.

Wilson W, Laidler P (1990) How teams can achieve 'skill blend'. Speech Therapy in Practice December, 7–8.

Wirz S (1993) Historical considerations in assessment. In Beech J, Harding L, Hilton-Jones D. (eds), Assessment in Speech and Language Therapy. London: Routledge.

Wirz S (1995) Perceptual Approaches to Communication Disorders. London: Whurr.

Wirz S, Beck J (1995) Assessment of voice quality: the Vocal Profiles Analysis Scheme. In Wirz S (ed.), Perceptual Approaches to Communication Disorders. London: Whurr.

Wootton A (1989) Speech to and from a severely retarded young Down's syndrome child. In Beveridge M, Conti-Ramsden G, Leudar I (eds), Language and Communication in Mentally Handicapped People. London: Chapman and Hall.

World Health Organization (1979) Health for All by the Year 2000. Global strategy from 32nd World Health Assembly. Geneva: WHO.

World Health Organization (1980) International Classification of Impairments, Disabilities and Handicaps (ICIDH). Geneva: WHO.

Wywialowski E (1993) Managing Client Care. St Louis: Mosby.

# Appendix
# Useful resources

The following list is taken from the text and also includes some additional sources of information. We hope it will allow easier access to some of the books we have mentioned. We acknowledge that there are numerous resources that we have not listed, the ones below are merely a starting point.

## General professional area

College of Speech and Language Therapists (1993) Audit: A Manual for Speech and Language Therapists. London: College of Speech and Language Therapists.

Department for Education (1994) Code of Practice on the Identification and Assessment of Special Educational Needs. London: Department for Education.

Enderby P, Emerson J (1995) Does Speech and Language Therapy Work? A Review of the Literature. London: Whurr.

Enderby P, John A (1997) Therapy Outcome Measures (Speech and Language Therapy). London: Singular Press.

Friel J (1997) Children with Special Needs: Assessment, Law and Practice – Caught in the Acts, 4th edn. London: Jessica Kingsley.

Hawkins P, Shohet R (1992) Supervision in the Helping Professions. Buckingham: Open University Press.

Health Service Journal.

Hegde MN (1987) Clinical Research in Communicative Disorders. Austin, Texas: pro-ed.

Royal College of Speech and Language Therapists (1996) Communicating Quality 2: Professional Standards for Speech and Language Therapists. London: RCSLT.

Sharkey P ( 1995) Introducing Community Care. London: Collins Educational.

Upton T, Brooks B (1995) Managing Change in the NHS. London: Kogan Page.

Worthington A (1993) Glossary of Syndromes Associated with Learning Difficulty. Manchester: Manchester Free Press.

## Assessment

Beech J, Harding L, Hilton-Jones D (eds) (1993) Assessment in Speech and Language Therapy. London: Routledge.

Crystal D (1992) Profiling Linguistic Disability, 2nd edn. London: Whurr.

Crystal D, Fletcher P, Garman M (1989) Grammatical Analysis of Language Disability, 2nd edn. London: Whurr.

Dodd B (1995) Differential Diagnosis and Treatment of Children with Speech Disorder. London: Whurr.

Edwards JA, Lampert MD (eds) (1993) Talking Data: Transcription and Coding in Discourse Research. Hillsdale, NJ: Lawrence Erlbaum.

Lees J, Urwin S (1997) Children with Language Disorders, 2nd edn. London: Whurr.

McDaniel D, McKee C, Smith Cairns H (1996) Methods for Assessing Children's Syntax. Cambridge, MA: MIT Press.

Miller J (1981) Assessing Language Production in Children. Baltimore: University Park Press.

Perkins M, Howard S (1995) Case Studies in Clinical Linguistics. London: Whurr.

Stackhouse J, Wells B (1997) Children's Speech and Literacy Problems: A psycholinguistic framework. London: Whurr.

Wirz S (1995) Perceptual Approaches to Communication Disorders. London: Whurr.

# Therapy

Barker P (1996) Basic Family Therapy, 3rd edn. London: Collins.

Beukelman DR, Yorkston KM, Dowden PA (1985) Communication Augmentation: A Casebook of Clinical Management. San Diego: College-Hill Press.

Chapey R (ed.) (1981) Language Intervention Strategies in Adult Aphasia. Baltimore: Williams & Wilkins.

Dalton P, Dunnett G (1992) A Psychology for Living: Personal Construct Theory for Professionals and Clients. Chichester: John Wiley and Sons.

Davis GA, Wilcox MJ (1985) Adult Aphasia Rehabilitation: Applied Pragmatics. Windsor: NFER-Nelson.

Dryden W (1990) Individual Therapy: A Handbook. Milton Keynes: Open University Press.

Duncan D (ed.) (1989) Working with Bilingual Language Disability. London: Chapman and Hall.

Fawcus M (ed.) (1992) Group Encounters in Speech and Language Therapy. Kibworth: Far Communications.

Grundy K (ed.) (1995) Linguistics in Clinical Practice, 2nd edn. London: Whurr.

Houghton D, McColgan M (1995) Working with Children. London: Collins Educational.

Howell J, Dean E (1994) Treating Phonological Disorders in Children: Metaphon – Theory to Practice, 2nd edn. London: Whurr.

Leahy M (ed.) (1989) Disorders of Communication: the Science of Intervention. London: Taylor and Francis.

Martin S (1987) Working with Dysphonics. Oxon: Winslow Press.

Rustin L, Cook F, Spence R (1995) The Management of Stuttering in Adolescence: A Communication Skills Approach. London: Whurr.

Selekman M (1993) Pathways to Change: Brief Therapy Solutions with Difficult Adolescents. New York/London: The Guilford Press.

Snowling M, Stackhouse J (eds) (1996) Dyslexia, Speech and Language: A Practitioner's Handbook. London: Whurr.

Street E (1994) Counselling for Family Problems. London: Sage.

# Useful INTERNET addresses

ACE centre – http://www.rmplc.co.uk/orgs/acecent/homepage.hmtl

ACE/ACCESS Centre – http://dspace.dial.pipex.com/town/terrace/ac969/

American Speech-Language-Hearing Association – http://www.asha.org/
DFEE Home Page – http://www.open.gov.uk/dfee/dfeehome.htm
Disability Net – http://dspace.dial.pipex.com/town/terrace/ac969/
Family Village – http://www.familyvillage.wise.edu/
National Association of Health Authorities and Trusts (NAHAT) – http://www.nahat.net/
Royal College of Speech and Language Therapists – http://www.rcslt.org
SCOPE – http://www.futurenet.co.uk/charity/scope/index.html
National Centre to Improve Practice in Special Education (NCIP) – http://www.edc.org/
    FSC/NCIP/

## Other useful addresses

Action for all Speech Impaired Children (AFASIC): 347 Central Markets, Smithfield,
    London EC1A 9NH
Aphasia – Action for Dysphasic Adults (ADA): 1 Royal Street, London SE1 7LL
Autism – National Autistic Society: 393 City Road, London EC1V 1NE
Carers – National Carers Association: 20–25 Glasshouse Yard, London EC1A 4JS
Communications Forum – PO Box 854, 3 Dufferin Street, London EC1Y 8NB
Disablement Information and Advice Line (DIAL UK) Park Lodge, St Catherine's
    Hospital, Tickhill Road, Doncaster, South Yorkshire DN4 8QN
Down's Syndrome Association: 155 Mitcham Road, Tooting, London SW17 9PG
Foundation for Communication for the Disabled (FCD): 25 High Street, Woking,
    Surrey, GU21 1BW
Independent Panel for Special Education Advice (IPSEA): 22 Warren Hill Road,
    Woodbridge, Suffolk IP12 4DU
Invalid Children's Aid Nationwide (I-CAN): Barbican Citygate, 1–3 Dufferin Street,
    London EC1Y 8NA
IN TOUCH Trust: 10 Norman Road, Sale, Cheshire M33 3DF
Makaton Vocabulary Development Project: 31 Firwood Drive, Camberley, Surrey GU15
    3QD
National Deaf-Blind and Rubella Association (Sense): 11–13 Clifton Terrace, London
    N4 3SR
Parent Network: 44–46 Caversham Road, London NW5 2DS
Royal National Institute for the Blind (RNIB): 224 Great Portland Street, London W1N
    6AA
Royal National Institute for Deaf People (RNID): 105 Gower Street, London WC1E 6AH
SCOPE: 16 Fitzroy Square, London W1P 4HQ
Stammering – British Stammering Association: 15 Old Ford Road, London E2 9PJ
Stroke Association: CHSA House, Whitecross Street, London EC1Y 8JJ

# Index

AAC 133
acquired disorder 4, 131
adolescence 130
advocacy 7
administrative staff 153, 162
Adult Training Centre 178
aims 49, 51, 98–99, 111, 113, 114, 118, 121
  long term 98
  short term 98
assessment 32, 33, 167, 221
  descriptive 33
  formal 35, 56
  informal 35, 56
  initial considerations 55, 56
  practice 32
  prescriptive 33
  process 32, 36
  screening 34
assistants 150–52, 183
ASTIIP 184
attention 47
attitudes 11
audit 212

bias
  clinical 54
  in data analysis 63
bilingual co-worker 152

carers 127, 223
care management 176, 180
care plans 176, 188
case history
  communication and language 45

development 42
medical 40
social/emotional 43–45
case records 187
change 7–15
  model of 125
  levels 125
  stages 16, 125
    action 17
    contemplation 16
    maintenance 16, 17
    pre-contemplation 16
charities 178, 183
Children Act 127, 157
Child Development Centre 145, 157
child protection 180
  co-ordinator 173
  process creativity 181
  register 180
  team 133, 139
child surveillance 159
classroom
  work within 168
client 2, 3
client centred approach 6, 7
clinical bias 54
clinical director 155, 160
clinical medical officer 174
Code of Practice 134, 164, 165, 167
coding 66
cognitive skills 47
collaboration 134, 135, 145
collating of information 71
communicative competence 68
Community Care Act 175

224

holistic approach 5
home 128, 157
home care worker 180
hospitals 154
hypothesis
    generation and testing 9, 72–74

impairment 23, 24
Individual Education Plan (IEP) 167,
    168
Individual Performance Review (IPR)
    206
Individual Program Plan (IPP) 177
induction
inductive thinking 32
information gathering 38
    direct 39
    indirect 39
    models 40, 41
information systems 198
initial contact 47–54
    closings 52
    openings 50
in patients 155
interdisciplinary 135
Internet 130, 222
intervention 12–31
    direct 26
    group 29
    indirect 27
    individual 28
    intensive 30
    models of 20
interpersonal skills 93
in touch 130, 223
INSET 170
institutionalisation 155
instrumental measures 62

journals 208

key worker 180
knowledge 10
    in therapy 90–92, 109, 125, 145

language 42
    comprehension 58-59
    content 46

elicitation 57
encouraging 57
form 46
sample 56
use 46
leadership 95, 139, 140
learning disability 166, 188
    team 133
literacy 46, 171
Local Management of Schools (LMS)
    163
locum agencies 185

maintenance
mainstream school 164
management 6
    clinical
    materials 103
medical information 40, 44
    records 187
memory 47
mental health 78
mentoring 203
methods 50, 51, 101, 102, 116
multi-disciplinary 132, 135, 144
    assesment 157

National Curriculum 163, 167
negotiation 141, 166
NHS, 134, 154
New NHS 159
non directive 91
non-organic causes 78
normalisation 176
nurse
    charge 160
    community 161
    district 161
    practice 161
    primary 160
    school 174
nurseries 179

objectives 50, 51, 99, 111, 113, 114,
    116, 119, 122
occupational therapy 147, 161, 182
OFSTED 163
organic causes 77

# DATE DUE